Infectious Causes of Cancer

Dedication

To my wife Liz and my son Ian

Infectious Causes of Cancer

A guide for nurses and healthcare professionals

Kenneth Campbell, MSc (Clinical Oncology)

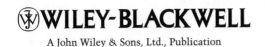

WILEY-BLACKWELL

A John Wiley & Sons, Ltd., Publication

This edition first published 2011
© 2011 John Wiley & Sons Ltd

Wiley-Blackwell is an imprint of John Wiley & Sons Ltd, formed by the merger of Wiley's global Scientific, Technical and Medical business with Blackwell Publishing Ltd.

Registered Office
John Wiley & Sons Ltd, The Atrium, Southern Gate, Chichester,
West Sussex, PO19 8SQ, United Kingdom

Editorial Offices
John Wiley & Sons Ltd, The Atrium, Southern Gate, Chichester, West Sussex,
PO19 8SQ, United Kingdom
9600 Garsington Road, Oxford, OX4 2DQ, United Kingdom
2121 State Avenue, Ames, Iowa 50014-8300, USA

For details of our global editorial offices, for customer services and for information about how to apply for permission to reuse the copyright material in this book please see our website at www.wiley.com/wiley-blackwell.

The right of the author to be identified as the author of this work has been asserted in accordance with the UK Copyright, Designs and Patents Act 1988.

Wiley publishes its books in a variety of electronic formats: ePDF 9780470753644.

Designations used by companies to distinguish their products are often claimed as trademarks. All brand names and product names used in this book are trade names, service marks, trademarks or registered trademarks of their respective owners. The publisher is not associated with any product or vendor mentioned in this book. This publication is designed to provide accurate and authoritative information in regard to the subject matter covered. It is sold on the understanding that the publisher is not engaged in rendering professional services. If professional advice or other expert assistance is required, the services of a competent professional should be sought.

Library of Congress Cataloging-in-Publication Data

Campbell, Ken, FIBMS.
  Infectious causes of cancer: a guide for nurses and healthcare professionals / Kenneth Campbell.
    p. ; cm.
  Includes bibliographical references and index.
  ISBN 978-0-470-51805-2 (pbk. : alk. paper) 1. Microbial carcinogenesis. 2. Viral carcinogenesis.
3. Cancer–Nursing. I. Title.
  [DNLM: 1. Neoplasms–etiology. 2. Neoplasms–nursing. 3. DNA Viruses–pathogenicity.
4. Nursing Care. 5. Oncogenic Viruses–pathogenicity.   WY 156]
  RC268.57.C357 2011
  616.99'401–dc22

                                            2010031090

A catalogue record for this book is available from the British Library.

Set in 10/12.5pt Palatino by SPi Publisher Services, Pondicherry, India
Printed and bound in Singapore by Markono Print Media Pte Ltd.

1   2011

Contents

Preface

Worldwide, over 10 million people are diagnosed with cancer each year and about 6 million people die each year of cancer; in the developing world as much as 25% of the cancer burden results from chronic infection[1]. Vaccination against Hepatitis B virus has had striking success in reducing the incidence of liver cancer in populations where the infection is endemic. Development of a vaccine against Human Papilloma Virus (HPV) offers hope of similar reduction in cervical cancer incidence.

This book, aimed principally at nurses and other healthcare professionals, will consider the epidemiology and biology of infectious causes of cancer. It will discuss each of the infectious agents associated with an increased risk of cancer discussing epidemiology of the infection and cancer(s), pathophysiology of the cancer(s) mechanisms, associated risk factors, and prevention of the infection and of the associated cancer(s).

It is vital for nurses and other healthcare professionals to be aware of the extent of infection-associated cancer and of how they can contribute to prevention of such cancers. Although the burden of infection-associated cancers is greatest in the developing world, they constitute a very significant fraction of all cases seen globally and the rise in global travel requires nurses to have a global understanding of health risks.

Reference

1. Bray, F. I. & Ferlay, J. (2003) The global burden of cancer. In: *World Cancer Report*, 1st edn (eds B. W. Stewart & P. Kleihues), pp. 11–19. IARC, Lyon.

Abbreviations

ABC	Abstain, Be faithful, use a Condom
AIDS	Acquired immune deficiency syndrome
ATLL	Adult T cell leukaemia/lymphoma
BBV	Blood-borne viruses
BCE	Before Christian Era
BL	Burkitt's Lymphoma
CAH	Chronic active hepatitis
CDC	Centers for Disease Control
CIN	Cervical intra-epithelial neoplasm
CKS	Classic Kaposi sarcoma
CMV	Cytomegalovirus
CTL	Cytotoxic T lymphocyte
CTVT	Canine transmissible venereal tumour
EBV	Epstein–Barr virus
ECC	Extrahepatic cholangiocarcinoma
ERV	Endogenous retrovirus
GBV	Hepatitis G virus
GERD	Gastro-oesophageal reflux disorder
GSHV	Ground squirrel hepatitis virus
GvHD	Graft versus host disease
HAART	Highly active anti-retroviral therapy
HAM/TSP	HTLV-1-associated myelopathy/Tropical spastic paresis
HBV	Hepatitis B virus
HCC	Hepatocellular carcinoma
HCV	Hepatitis C virus
HDV	Hepatitis D virus
HER	Human endogenous retrovirus
HGV	Hepatitis G virus
HHMMTV	Human homologue of MMTV
HHV4	Human herpesvirus 4
HHV8	Human herpesvirus 8
HIV	Human immunodeficiency virus
HL	Hodgkin Lymphoma

HNC	Head and neck cancer
HNSCC	Squamous cell carcinoma of the head and neck
HPA	Health Protection Agency
HPV	Human papillomavirus
HSV	Herpes simplex virus
HTLV-1	Human T lymphotropic virus-1
	Human T cell leukaemia virus-1
IAC	Infection-associated cancer
IARC	International Agency for Research on Cancer
ICC	Intrahepatic cholangiocarcinoma
IM	Infectious mononucleosis
IP-CNS	Immunoblastic primary central nervous system lymphoma
KS	Kaposi sarcoma
KSHV	Kaposi sarcoma-associated herpesvirus
LSHTM	London School of Hygiene and Tropical Medicine
MALT	Mucosa-associated lymphoid tissue
MALToma	Mucosa-associated lymphoid tissue lymphoma
MCC	Merkel cell carcinoma
MCD	Multi-centric Castleman's disease
MCPV	Merkel cell polyomavirus
MCV	Merkel cell virus
MMTV	Murine mammary tumour virus
MSM	Men who have sex with men
NAT	Nucleic acid test
NPC	Nasopharyngeal carcinoma
PEL	Primary effusion lymphoma
PMTCT	Prevention of mother to child transmission
PTLD	Post-transplant lymphoproliferative disorder
PWHA	People with HIV or AIDS
QALY	Quality adjusted life year
RSV	Rous sarcoma virus
SABC	Schistosomiasis-associated bladder cancer
SCC	Squamous cell carcinoma
SSE	Stratified squamous epithelium
STI	Sexually transmitted infection
SV40	Simian virus 40
TCC	Transitional cell carcinoma
TRIM	Transfusion-related immunomodulation
TTI	Transfusion-transmitted infection
VLP	Virus-like particle
WHO	World Health Organization
WHV	Woodchuck hepatitis virus

Introduction

Over 99% of the world's population is infected with at least one potentially cancer-causing organism. Clearly, the mere presence of such an organism is not typically sufficient to cause cancer – in most, and probably all, cases the infection is a *necessary* but not *sufficient* cause[1]. Fortunately, the requirement for cofactors ensures that most such infections only cause cancer in a small proportion of infected individuals. Despite this, infections are estimated collectively to account for at least 16% of all cancers globally, while in the developing world the proportion may be greater than 20%[2]. Kinlen has pointed out that these are likely to be underestimates since they do not include instances of infections acting as co-carcinogens[3], while Blattner has suggested that viruses alone may account for 20% of all cancers[4]. It is often stated that cervical cancer is unique in always being associated with a specific causal agent (human papillomavirus (HPV) which has been demonstrated in 99.7% of cervical cancer specimens examined[5]); this is not strictly true since the presence of HTLV-1 is part of the definition of Adult T cell leukaemia/lymphoma (ATTL)[6]. It is clear that, although HPV infection is necessary for cervical cancer to develop, it is not sufficient; if it were, the incidence of cervical cancer would be much higher, it is the second commonest cancer affecting women globally and, in some developing countries it is the most common female cancer. It has been suggested that 'Most women in the world are probably infected with at least one if not several types of HPV during their sexual life.'[7]

Throughout most of human history, conditions of hygiene and sanitation now seen only in the developing world and amongst the very poor were the norm. This implies that the global impact of infectious causes of cancer would almost certainly have been significantly greater than in modern times. Many of the commoner cancers in the developed world are diseases of late life so they are comparatively rare in populations with short average life expectancy. This has led some writers to claim that pre-industrial societies enjoy immunity from cancer; more careful studies have shown that *age-adjusted* rates are usually comparable to global rates. The greatest potentially avoidable cause of cancer is, of course, cigarette smoking – unfortunately, it has proved very difficult to change smoking

Infectious Causes of Cancer, first edition. By Ken Campbell. Published 2011 by John Wiley & Sons Ltd.
© 2011 John Wiley & Sons Ltd.

habits at the population level. It is clear that cigarette smoking is a cofactor increasing the risk of several types of infection-associated cancer, including cervical cancer and gastric cancer[8,9].

The chief contributors to the burden of infection-associated cancer are *Helicobacter pylori* (gastric cancer and lymphoma)[10], human papillomaviruses (cervical and other cancers)[11] and the hepatitis B virus (hepatocellular carcinoma)[12]; together these are estimated to account for over 90% of infection-associated cancers[2]. The most ubiquitous of the cancer-causing infections is Epstein-Barr virus (EBV), which is estimated to infect around 95% of the global adult population; in most cases the virus is acquired during childhood and is asymptomatic throughout life[13]. Although EBV is near universal in distribution it is most frequently associated with malignant transformation in immunocompromised individuals.

Several other virus species are known to cause cancer, as well as parasites which, although rare in the developed world, are common in areas of South-East Asia. Although these parasites are rare in the developed world, knowledge of the associated clinical conditions is necessary as the associated cancers may be encountered in any clinical environment. In many cases the infestation can be acquired by very brief exposure and so tourists may be vulnerable, also the scale of population movement and the long latency between infestation and cancer diagnosis mean that patients may have spent many years living in the developed world before being diagnosed with a parasite-linked cancer. In addition to those infectious organisms definitely identified as causes of specific cancers, there are others which are suspected of carcinogenic potential.

There are various pathways by which infection may lead to cancer. In virtually all cases there is an extended latency – sometimes decades long – between initial infection and eventual diagnosis of cancer; there are a few exceptions to this principle such as childhood endemic Burkitt's lymphoma. Carcinogenesis may be direct, for example by insertion of viral genes into the cell's genome triggering malignant transformation; or it may be indirect, for example by induction of chronic inflammation (cirrhosis, chronic gastritis) which creates a local environment with a greatly increased risk of transformation occurring, or when the infective organism suppresses the host immune response.

Commonly, only a small percentage of infected individuals develop cancer – in the case of *Helicobacter pylori*, India has one of the highest infection rates in the world but the incidence of gastric cancer is low[14]. The risk of gastric cancer in *Helicobacter pylori* carriers appears to be determined by a combination of host factors (host genetics), bacterial factors (bacterial genetics) and environmental factors (diet, smoking, etc.)[15]. In some cases the infection appears to be a necessary, albeit not sufficient, cause of the cancer; perhaps the most striking example of this is high-risk human papillomavirus (HPV) and cancer of the uterine cervix[5].

The proportion of cancer with an infectious aetiology is greatest in the developing world but, even in the developed world, infection-associated cancers constitute a high proportion of the potentially preventable cancers. The example of the vaccines being introduced to clinical use to prevent infection with high-risk human papillomaviruses offer a paradigm. Successful implementation of a programme of vaccination will require cooperation between public health officials and nurses working in primary care, sexual health and health education. It will also require collaboration with professionals working with young people in arenas such as teaching, social work and professional youth workers. There are already indications that some groups, often but not always with religious affiliations, are opposing vaccination on the grounds that sexual chastity provides complete protection and that vaccination of young girls (the primary target group) will encourage under-age sexual activity. Successful challenges to these obstacles offers a future in which the Pap smear is seen as a 'back-up' precaution with very low levels of positive smears. Failure to meet the challenges would mean that women continue to die from a highly preventable form of cancer.

Reduction of the burden of infection-associated cancer will require a combination of primary prevention (blocking transmission of infection, boosting host immune resistance by vaccination), and secondary prevention (preventing progression from chronic infection to malignant transformation). In the case of hepatitis B there is compelling evidence that infection during early infancy carries a high risk of eventual cancer, while infection in adult life confers a much lower risk – clearly the priority here must be to prevent mother to child transmission. Cervical cancer, as already described, is a consequence of infection with high-risk HPV strains; in almost all cases infection is acquired early after a woman becomes sexually active. This process is best prevented by ensuring vaccination before young women first experience penetrative sex. A number of tropical infections, such as schistosomiasis and fluke infections appear to be potentially carcinogenic at whatever age they are acquired, and this requires programmes to interrupt transmission between human hosts. It is likely to take decades, at least, before any of these cancer pathways is effectively blocked, so nurses and other healthcare professionals continue to require a knowledge and understanding of the nature of infection-associated cancers.

References

1. Fischinger, P.J. (1992) Prospects for reducing virus-associated human cancers by antiviral vaccines. *Journal of National Cancer Institute. Monographs*, **12**, 109–114.

2. Pisani, P., Parkin, D.M., Munoz, N. & Ferlay, J. (1997) Cancer and infection: Estimates of the attributable fraction in 1990. *Cancer Epidemiology, Biomarkers and Prevention*, **6**, 387–340.

3. Kinlen, L. (2004) Infections and immune factors in cancer: The role of epidemiology. *Oncogene*, **23**, 6341–6348.

4. Blattner, W.A. (1999) Human retroviruses: their role in cancer. *Proceedings of the Association of American Physicians*, **111**, 563–572.

5. Walboomers, J.M., Jacobs, M.V., Manos, M.M., Bosch, F.X., Kummer, J.A. & Shah, K.V. (1999) Human papillomavirus is a necessary cause of invasive cervical cancer worldwide. *Journal of Pathology*, **189**, 12–19.

6. Takatsuki, K. (2005) Discovery of adult T-cell leukemia. *Retrovirology*, **2**, 17.

7. Schiffman, M., Castle, P.E., Jeronimo, J., Rodriguez, A.C. & Wacholder, S. (2007) Human papillomavirus and cervical cancer. *Lancet*, **370**, 890–907.

8. Quinn, M. (2005) Cervix. In: *Cancer Atlas of the United Kingdom and Ireland 1991–2000* (eds Quinn, M., Wood, H., Cooper, N. & Rowan, S.), pp. 71–78. Palgrave Macmillan, Basingstoke.

9. Steward, J. & Wood, H. (2005) Stomach. In: *Cancer Atlas of the United Kingdom and Ireland 1991–2000* (eds Quinn, M., Wood, H., Cooper, N. & Rowan, S.), pp. 219–229. Palgrave Macmillan, Basingstoke.

10. Ahmed, N. & Sechi, L.A. (2005) *Helicobacter pylori* and gastroduodenal pathology: New threats of the old friend. *Annals of Clinical Microbiology and Antimicrobials*, **4** (1), 1.

11. zur Hausen, H. (2002) Papillomaviruses and cancer: From basic studies to clinical application. *Nature Reviews. Cancer*, **2**, 342–350.

12. McGlynn, K.A. & London, W.T. (2005) Epidemiology and natural history of hepatocellular carcinoma. *Best Practice & Research. Clinical Gastroenterology*, **19**, 3–23.

13. Andersson, J. (2000) An overview of Epstein-Barr virus: From discovery to future directions for treatment and prevention. *Herpes*, **7**, 76–82.

14. Prabhu, S.R., Amrapurkar, A.D. & Amrapurkar, D.N. (1995) Role of *Helicobacter pylori* in gastric carcinoma. *The National Medical Journal of India*, **8**, 58–60.

15. Megraud, F. & Lehours, P. (2004) *Helicobacter pylori* and gastric cancer prevention is possible. *Cancer Detection and Prevention*, **28**, 392–398.

1 Historical background

Although cancer is described in ancient manuscripts, it is only in the last 150 years that there has been clear recognition of the nature of the disease. At the end of the eighteenth century, cancer was widely believed to be contagious; not until the early twentieth century did clear evidence begin to emerge that cancer, while not itself infectious, may be caused by infectious organisms. As we enter the twenty-first century, there is sufficient understanding of infection-associated cancer to allow ambitious prophylaxis schemes to be undertaken.

Antiquity of cancer

It is probable that cancer has existed for hundreds of millions of years, since the emergence of the first complex multicellular organisms. In a multicelled organism it is vital for cell growth and division to be tightly regulated; indeed cancer can be defined as a breakdown of the regulation of cell growth, division and death. There are reliable descriptions of malignant tumours in modern invertebrates, implying that cancer antedated the emergence of vertebrates.

In fossilized bones, in contrast, it is often possible to delineate very fine details of internal structure and, in some cases, evidence of erosion caused by soft tissue swellings; some bones show changes consistent with specific cancers, or bone metastases[1]. There is a general consensus that there is physical evidence of malignant disease in dinosaurs. Fossilized remains of a caterpillar from over 20 million years ago have been found to contain tumours which may have been caused by viral infection[2].

Plant tumours such as crown galls have been compared with animal cancers[3,4]; it has been known for a century that one of the commonest causes of such growths is a bacterial infection – *Agrobacterium tumefaciens*[5].

Infectious Causes of Cancer, first edition. By Ken Campbell. Published 2011 by John Wiley & Sons Ltd.
© 2011 John Wiley & Sons Ltd.

The Kanam mandible

The Kanam mandible is a jawbone fragment from an early hominid, who is esti-mated to have lived between 500 000 and 1 million years ago; it was discovered by Louis Leakey in Kenya in the 1930s[6]. The inner surface of the jawbone bears a tumour mass often cited as the oldest example of a human cancer. Some have sug-gested it to be an osteogenic sarcoma, others consider it to be a Burkitt lymphoma (BL)[7] (a tumour associated in sub-Saharan Africa with Epstein–Barr virus infec-tion). Unfortunately however a recent re-examination using sophisticated technol-ogy concluded that '...*both macro and microanatomy are consistent with bone pathology secondary to fracture*'[8]. It would seem that the unfortunate owner of the Kanam mandible suffered not cancer but a broken jaw. There is no obvious candidate to replace the Kanam mandible as the oldest known hominid cancer. Many prehis-toric bony remains bear probable tumours but none has an unequivocal hallmark of cancer. Stathopoulos, in a book chapter on 'Bone tumours in antiquity'[9] lists many of these. Newby and Howard state '*The oldest specimen of a human cancer was found in a female skull dating from the Bronze Age (1900–1600 BCE)*'[10]; unfortunately they give no source to support this assertion.

The cancer papyruses

The oldest written descriptions of cancer are found in Egyptian papyruses which date to around 1500 BCE and are based on tracts from around 2500 BCE. Many elements of the papyri are difficult to interpret, due to changed terminology and disease concepts. The Edwin Smith papyrus describes surgical cases; at least one case seems to be a cancer (of the breast)[11]. The papyruses are purely case histories with no speculation as to causes of cancer. It is probable that, like other natural phenomena in the prescience era, they attributed development of cancer to super-natural causes.

Graeco-Roman literature

Hippocrates (460–375 BCE) is credited with the first use of the term cancer (Gk crab)[12]; possibly because the growths reminded him of a moving crab. He used the terms '*carcinos (a tumor), carcinoma (a malignant tumor) and cancer (a non-healing malignant ulcer)*'[13]. Hippocrates believed that severe, incurable and ulcerated cancers arose from an excess of black bile, while thin bile was responsible for non-ulcerated, curable cancers.

The first specific text on tumours was Galen's 'De Tumoribus Praeter Naturam' (Tumours contrary to nature)[14] written almost 2000 years ago. To Galen, tumours meant all swellings, including conditions such as dropsy and even obesity. He embraced the Hippocratic 'humoral' theory of the nature of disease, including cancer – unfortunately for the next 1500 years no one successfully challenged anything written by Galen. In 1543, Vesalius, Professor of Anatomy at Padua, was the first to seriously challenge Galen's errors on anatomy[15] ushering in a new understanding of anatomy; unfortunately Galen's humoral theory of disease continued to hold sway. Vesalius also *'wrestled with the knotty problem of clinical differentiation of tumours'*[16]. Physicians in the late sixteenth century did not differentiate clearly between neoplastic growths and other forms of swelling, thus Benoît (translated by Hunton) wrote, *'Every Cancer almost is uncurable, or hardly cured, sith it is indeede a particular and worst kind of Leprosie'*[17].

Humours, tumours and cell theories

In 1700, Deshaies Gendron published a closely reasoned argument that cancers were not *'inflammatory masses composed of fluted humours'* but rather solid structures composed of body tissues and capable of destructive growth[18]. In clear contradiction of Galen's teachings, he based this on *'clinical studies and observations of cancerous materials'*[19]. Sadly, the dead hand of Galen lay heavy and Gendron's work was rejected and lay forgotten for many years. It was to be more than a century before medicine emphatically discarded the humoral theory.

At the end of the eighteenth century, cancer was widely thought to be an infectious disease; because of which the first cancer hospital in France (opened in 1779) was forced to move from the city. This was largely influenced by two seventeenth-century clinicians, who argued from analogy to other 'tumours' such as leprosy and elephantiasis – both of which are transmissible[16]. Beckett, writing in 1712, explicitly rejected the analogy between cancer and elephantiasis, declaring that *'tho' a Cancer has some similitude to an Elephantiasis, they are different Diseases'*[20].

Cancer patients continued to be refused admission to many hospitals as late as the mid-nineteenth century. Records of the Women's Hospital in New York show that the Board of Lady Supervisors refused admission of cancer patients to the hospital 'pavilions' – clearly due to a belief that all growths, including cancer, were contagious. The surgeon Marion Sims challenged the Board head-on and continued to admit, and operate upon, patients with early stage cancer. Unfortunately, the result was Sims's dismissal; he went on to become President of the American Medical Association[21], so this contretemps clearly did not permanently blight his career.

Reports of 'cancer houses' persisted into the twentieth century and there are still many people who fear that cancer itself is infectious. Alternative explanations exist for multiple cases at a given address; familial cancers may have affected several related occupants of the same dwelling, there may have been shared exposures to environmental carcinogens or there may have been transmission within families of organisms like *Helicobacter pylori* which are known to increase cancer risk.

At the commencement of the nineteenth century with the flourishing of scientific medicine there was a great deal of interest in the nature, causes and treatment of cancer. In 1800/1801, French anatomist Marie François Xavier Bichat *'laid down the principles that all tissue was similar in structure, that each type of tissue was a unit of life capable of reproducing itself, and that tumours, cicatrices (scars) and cysts were not inflammations but an overgrowth of cellular tissue'*[19]; like Gendron, Bichat appears to have been far ahead of his time; it was to be more than 50 years before Virchow published his famous axiom *'omnis cellula e cellula'* – all cells arise from existing cells[22].

In 1802, in London, a group of prominent physicians and lay people formed the "Institution for Investigating the Nature and Cure of Cancer"[23]. They formulated a list of 13 key questions, most of which are as relevant today as when they were formulated two centuries ago:

(1) What are the diagnostic signs of cancer?

(2) Does any alteration take place in the structure of a part, preceding that more obvious change which is called cancer? If there does, what is the nature of that alteration?

(3) Is cancer always an original and primary disease, or may other diseases degenerate into cancer?

(4) Are there any proofs of cancer being a hereditary disease?

(5) Are there any proofs of cancer being a contagious disease?

(6) Is there any well-marked relation between cancer and other diseases? If there be, what are those diseases to which it bears the nearest resemblance, in its origin, progress and termination?

(7) May cancer be regarded at any period, or under any circumstances, merely as a local disease? Or, does the existence of cancer in one part, afford a presumption, that there is a tendency to a similar morbid alteration in other parts of the animal system?

(8) Has climate, or local situation, any influence in rendering the human constitution more or less liable to cancer, under any form, or in any part?

(9) Is there a particular temperament of body more liable to be affected with cancer than others? And if there be, what is that temperament?

(10) Are brute creatures subject to any disease, resembling cancer in the human subject?

(11) Is there any period of life absolutely exempt from the attack of this disease?

(12) Are the lymphatic glands ever affected primarily in cancer?

(13) Is cancer under any circumstances susceptible of a natural cure?

Theories other than contagion were put forward, perhaps the most prominent being the lymph theory and the blastema theory; the former suggested that cancers arose from local accumulations of lymph, the latter acknowledged that cancers were formed of cells but held that these arose from budding elements, blastema, found between normal cells. Rudolph Virchow argued correctly that all cells (including those in tumours) arise from existing tissues – 'omnis cellula e cellula' and also identified chronic inflammation as a mechanism of carcinogenesis; – one pathway by which infection can lead to malignant transformation. Virchow mistakenly believed that cancers *'spread like a liquid'*. Thomas Hodgkin, after whom

Hodgkin lymphoma is named, recognized that metastasis occurred by spread of elements of the original cancer; *'At the same time, I would by no means deny the possibility, or even probability, that some of the nucleated cells may find their way into the blood, and be arrested at particular parts, giving rise to productions similar to the original tumour, more especially when the latter has advanced to the softening stage, and the lymphatic glands have become affected'*[24].

From the late 1800s into the early twentieth century, both scientists and lay people believed that cancer could be initiated by a single local trauma (as opposed to chronic irritation). Despite the failure to induce tumours in animals by deliberate injury this belief was maintained and is still a popular folk explanation for the aetiology of cancer. It is probable that this was based, at least in part, on incidents when a tumour was first noticed following an injury close to its location.

The interval between the first recognition of the virus as a distinct biological entity and the first proposal that they might play a significant part in cancer causation was remarkably short[25]. In 1892, the first virus (tobacco mosaic) was identified by Ivanovsky, in 1898 foot-and-mouth disease became the first animal virus to be identified, by Loeffler and Frosch, while in 1901, yellow fever was the first human virus identified, by Reed; as early as 1903 Amédée Borrel proposed that viruses might be common causes of cancer[26]. In a little over a century not only was it established how important and widespread viruses are as human carcinogens, it was also research on cancer and viruses which led to *'the concept of the oncogene, the identification of the p53 tumor suppressor, and the function of the retinoblastoma tumor suppressor'*[25].

'False dawns' and delayed recognition

In 1910 Peyton Rous, working at the Rockefeller Institute in New York, reported *'the first avian tumor that has proved transplantable to other individuals'*[27]. Just one year later, Rous published the first experimental proof of transmission by a cell-free preparation of a malignant tumour[28]. In 1908, Ellerman and Bang had described similar experiments with transfer of avian leukaemia[29], indeed Rous made reference to their work in his 1910 paper – *'Ellerman and Bang have shown chicken leukemia to be transmissible, and in some of their animals aleukemic lymphomata resulted from inoculation. But they have also shown, as have Hirschfeld and Jaeoby, that the disease is dependent on a filterable virus.'* Prior to the 1930s, few researchers or clinicians regarded leukaemia as a malignant disease, so these seminal reports were not seen as relevant to cancer aetiology.

Many used a strangely circular logic to dispute the malignant nature of the tumours reported by Rous; they argued that as the tumours had been induced by an infectious agent and it was well known that infectious agents do not cause cancer the growths could not be malignant. Rous clearly anticipated this challenge as he states in his paper *'It is evident from the foregoing description that our tumor of the fowl possesses to a marked degree those characters of morphology and behavior which distinguish the true malignant neoplasms, especially the sarcomata'*[28]. An alternative, equally facile argument, was that filtration had been inadequate to remove all cell-fragments and that cells from an existing tumour had been transplanted[30, 31]. Many of those who did accept Rous's achievement still insisted that it had no relevance for humans, or indeed any mammals; they considered transmissibility to be a peculiar feature of avian tumours[32], without offering any rationale why this might be the case. Rous *et al.* went on to confirm their findings and to demonstrate that other avian tumours were transmissible in a similar fashion[33].

Rous carried out an unsuccessful search for mammalian tumour viruses – his failure led him to move away from work on infectious causes of cancer. Rous was eventually drawn back into researching viral oncogenesis in the early 1930s when Richard Shope published his findings on the induction of tumours in rabbits by papillomaviruses[34,35]. Those who were determined that infection played no part in the aetiology of human cancer deployed the same peculiar arguments used against Rous; some claimed that these could not be true cancers as they were caused by infection, while others conceded that this was proof that cancer could be transmissible in mammals but were insistent that this had no relevance for humans. Shope and Rous were to enter into a very productive collaboration – many of their discoveries are still central to understanding of viral induction of cancer. Rous's biography on the Nobel Prize website (www.nobelprize.org) describes him and Shope as friends as well as collaborators; despite this, they appear to have published no joint papers.

In 1926, there was a major stimulus to the notion of infection as a significant cause of cancer. A Nobel Prize was awarded to Johannes Fibiger for apparently demonstrating that a nematode worm caused stomach cancer in laboratory rats[36,37]. Fibiger, a Danish medical researcher, was studying tuberculosis in rats when he observed that three of his animals had developed stomach tumours. These appeared to be associated with the ingestion of nematodes present in cockroaches fed to the rats. In reality, the diet was the crucial factor; Fibiger's rats were vitamin A deficient, which has been shown to cause stomach cancer in mice[38–40], the nematodes were not involved in the cancer.

Fibiger's Nobel Prize is often said to have been awarded on the basis of a (subsequently disproved) claim that he had found the first infectious cause of cancer, yet his lecture makes it clear that he considered infection as a cause of cancer to be well established by the time of his key papers and that he, *correctly*, saw his key achievement as the development of a method to systematically induce tumours in animal studies. Researchers, including Fibiger, went on to use chemical agents to induce tumours in experimental models and the value of this to cancer research cannot be overstated. In his Nobel Prize lecture, Fibiger makes it clear that he believed that his results were associated with the specific nematode he had isolated from his animals, which he named *Spiroptera neoplastica*; however, he made no claim that this was the first evidence of infectious causes. In his Nobel lecture[41], Fibiger states

'...*Schizostomum hæmatobium's aetiological importance in the development of cancer of the bladder must be considered as proven. Nor can it be doubted that other Trematodes, such as Opisthorchis felineus, Schizostomum japonicum and Clonorchis sinensis can, in certain cases, bring about primary carcinoma of the liver, and that Schizostomum mansoni can be the cause of polyps and carcinoma in the colon.'* and later *'In the course of the research work on Spiroptera carcinoma, it became possible for the first time to induce typical, metastasizing carcinomas systematically and at will. This provided experimental proof that the start of a cancer can, in agreement with the theory of Virchow, be brought about by external, exogenic influences, and lent support to experiments on the effects of long-term irritants of other kinds'*[41].

Many agree that an unfortunate consequence of Fibiger's 'mistaken' Nobel award was the delay in official recognition of Peyton Rous's work on avian tumour viruses; Rous's belated award was the first in 40 years for cancer-related work. Peyton Rous was to eventually receive a Nobel Prize for his work, but not until 1966, just 4 years before he died[42]. Rous was dogmatic in rejecting the notion that genetic changes played any significant part in carcinogenesis; *'What can be the nature of the generality of neoplastic changes, the reason for their persistence, their irreversibility, and for the discontinuous, steplike alterations that they frequently undergo? A favorite explanation has been that oncogens cause alterations in the genes of the cells of the body, somatic mutations as these are termed. But numerous facts, when taken together, decisively exclude this supposition'*[43]. (Oncogens is the term Rous used for agents now know as carcinogens. It was perhaps fortunate that terminology changed since the scope for confusion with *oncogenes* is obvious.) It is, of course, now beyond dispute that cancer is essentially a genetic disorder – the lesion lies at the level of the DNA molecule and the observable tumour is a late consequence of a process that began with a single cell containing a corrupt copy of the genome[44].

The 1930s also saw John Bittner's studies on murine mammary tumours. It had been shown that certain strains of mice were prone to mammary cancers and that the strain of the male was irrelevant; if the female was from a tumour-prone strain all her female offspring would share this vulnerability[45]. Bittner carried out what proved to be the crucial experiment; newborn mice from high-risk females were suckled by low-risk females and vice versa. The risk of mammary cancer was high only where the newborn had received milk from a high-risk female[46]. By 1942, it had been established that this was due to passage of a virus[47]; this retrovirus is called the murine mammary tumour virus (MMTV)[48]. (Retroviruses, such as HIV, contain no DNA in their infective particles; their genome is coded in RNA and before they can replicate they must transcribe this into DNA, using an enzyme called reverse transcriptase.) For over 30 years there has been speculation that at least a proportion of cases of breast cancer may have a viral aetiology[49] and suspects include MMTV or a human homologue of this virus (HHMMTV), HPV and EBV[50].

Burkitt's great tumour safari

In 1958, Dennis Burkitt, a surgeon working for the Colonial Medical Service in Uganda, described the unusual tumour which still bears his name – Burkitt's lymphoma[51]. Having seen two cases in which children presented with strikingly symmetrical jaw tumours, Burkitt reviewed the records of 41 cases of children with jaw tumours and found histology available on 29 of these; in each case there were similar undifferentiated round cells – although he made clear his uncertainty of the nature of the tumour, he initially described it as a sarcoma. By 1958 Burkitt had written these cases up ~ within 2 years Burkitt, working with histopathologist Greg O'Conor, had determined they were of lymphoid origin[52,53].The 1961 papers were based on many more cases Burkitt identified by questionnaires and personal contact with physicians. Some remarkable features emerged; the tumour was very common in what Burkitt referred to as a 'lymphoma belt' which spanned the Equator roughly between 15° north and south with a tail extending south along the coast of east Africa[54].

It occurred in children of all tribes and ethnic backgrounds living in this region but not if they lived above 5000 ft above sea level; within the belt the new tumour was far more common than any other childhood cancer. In an attempt to explain this phenomenon, Burkitt set out upon what he termed a '*tumour safari*'[55]: a 10 000 mile journey along the southern edge of the lymphoma belt; Burkitt sought to identify what changed at the boundary. The key variable was temperature – below 5000 ft and within the lymphoma belt the minimum temperature did not fall below about 60°F (15.5°C). This suggested a mosquito-borne infection as the cause, and many possible causal agents were considered, including malaria. By chance, when Burkitt lectured in London in 1961, virologist Anthony Epstein was in the audience – he was intrigued by the possibility of a viral cause and arranged for frozen tumour samples to be sent to him at the Bland Sutton Institute[54].

In 1964 Epstein, with Bert Achong and Yvonne Barr, published a description of a new virus identified by electron microscopy of the samples[56]; which they named Epstein–Barr virus (after the cell-line from which it was isolated). Epstein describes facing a high level of scepticism[57], some refused to believe that the cells were lymphoid, and others that the particles were viruses. Electron microscopy was in its infancy and many believed the observations were of artefacts of tissue fixation and processing. Within 20 years, the EBV genome had been fully sequenced[58] – the first human virus for which this was achieved.

There was further reluctance to concede a causal link between EBV and human cancer. At first it was called a contaminant or a passenger, of cells perhaps made susceptible by early stages of malignant transformation. This led to the definitive International Agency for Research on Cancer (IARC) 7-year study of 42 000 children in Uganda's West Nile district[59]. EBV is now accepted as a key causal factor in 'endemic' or 'African' Burkitt's[60]; the disease is also seen in a 'sporadic' form as an AIDS-defining condition[61] and in non-immunosuppressed patients, but it was the endemic form which yielded the first known human cancer virus. For many years it has been accepted that when children with chronic immunosuppression, due to malaria infection, acquired EBV the lack of immune surveillance allowed the virus to multiply rapidly and induce BL. It has recently been suggested that malarial infection may play a more direct role in lymphomagenesis[62], and other even more complex mechanisms have been postulated, involving three different infections and a tumour promoter[63].

Other forms of immunosuppression can increase the risk of BL; it is classed as an AIDS-defining malignancy. There are now recognized to be three classes of BL[64]:

■ Endemic – African children, often with bilateral jaw lesions – almost 100% EBV+
■ Sporadic – seen in adults and children in all populations – minority EBV+
■ Immunodeficiency-related – mainly HIV-positive, but also transplant recipients and congenital immunodeficiency – most are EBV+

Stomach bugs Down Under

Scarcely more than 20 years ago, two Australian medical researchers transformed our understanding of the pathophysiology of gastric ulcers. They went on to demonstrate that infection with the bacterium *H. pylori* is a key factor in some forms of stomach cancer and of certain forms of lymphoma. Initially there was scepticism about the possibility of persistent gastric infection with any organism. This has been portrayed by some as rejection by entrenched interests of new ideas, but Atwood debunks this view[65].

Helicobacter spp. were first described as resident in the mammalian stomach in the late nineteenth century[66], being described as spiral-shaped bacteria in the stomachs of dogs – '*Even more exciting are certain spirilli I found constantly in the dog's stomach and that, in addition to being numerous in the mucus layer that covers the mucosa, penetrate into the gland lumen of both pylorus and fundus, and sometimes reach the bottom glands*'. The observation was dismissed as insignificant for many years; there was a consensus that the interior of the stomach had no resident microbial flora. This was the prevailing view when pathologist Robin Warren reported observing unidentified curved bacteria (*H. pylori*) on the gastric epithelium of patients with active chronic gastritis[67]. The following year, with gastroenterologist Barry Marshall, he published a paper on the association of this organism with gastritis and peptic ulceration. This paper eventually led to the award to Warren and Marshall of the Nobel Prize for Physiology or Medicine in 2006. Warren failed many times to culture the organism; standard practice was to discard cultures after 48h and success came by chance when, over Easter, a set of cultures was left in an incubator for 5 days[68]. Marshall famously attempted to satisfy Koch's postulates[69] – one of which requires that the agent be administered to a susceptible organism and induce the disease with which it is associated – by swallowing *H. pylori*, which induced gastritis but no ulcer or cancer[70,71]. Fortunately, there is now an animal model[72], so future researchers will be spared the gastric discomfort and extreme halitosis his experiment induced.

Previously stomach ulcers were ascribed to behavioural (and possibly genetic) factors. The archetypal ulcer victim was the highly stressed executive, with a non-stop life, too many lunchtime martinis and too much spicy food – 'hurry, worry and curry'. Treatment was either medical, with a bland diet, modified life-style, and antacids, or surgical, involving removal of all or part of the stomach. An acid blocking drug called Zantac, rapidly became the world's biggest selling prescription drug and ensured the fortunes of pharmaceutical company Glaxo. Use of inexpensive antibiotic regimens to eradicate *H. pylori* was found to heal the ulcers; unlike prior medical management, this was followed by very low rates of recurrence.

Marshall has claimed that after one *H. pylori* meeting in Chicago the fall in Glaxo's share price represented a reduction of about $1 billion in the company's value[65].

Within a decade of the Warren and Marshall paper, it had been established that *H. pylori* is a significant carcinogen. In 1994, following a review of the evidence, the IARC reported that *H. pylori* was classified as a carcinogen in humans[73]. It has been known since the time of Virchow that chronic inflammation is causally linked with cancer[74] and many assumed that this was the sole basis for the association between gastric ulcers and gastric cancers; more recent studies have demonstrated complex interactions at the genetic level which moderate immune responses and may directly stimulate malignant transformation[75].

Oncogenes, retroviruses and more Nobel Prizes

An understanding of malignant transformation depended on the flowering of molecular biology. Watson and Crick's description of the structure of DNA[76] was the first step on a road which has led to the deciphering of the human genome. A concept known as the 'central dogma'[77] states that DNA is transcribed to RNA which directs synthesis of proteins; RNA viruses (retroviruses) require an additional preliminary step in which they transcribe their RNA-encoded genome into DNA using the enzyme reverse transcriptase. In 1975, Baltimore, Dulbecco and Temin shared the Nobel Prize for *'their discoveries concerning the interaction between tumour viruses and the genetic material of the cell'* – essentially for the discovery of reverse transcriptase.

The avian leukaemia and sarcoma viruses discovered at the dawn of the twentieth century were retroviruses, although neither the term nor the concept existed at the time Ellerman and Bang and Rous were reporting their discoveries. In 1961, Crawford reported that Rous Sarcoma Virus contains RNA[78]; this led oncogenic retroviruses to be described as RNA tumour viruses.

Key concepts in the modern understanding of how a cancer develops are the oncogene and the tumour suppressor gene – these concepts are discussed in further detail in the next section. Oncogenes are significant in the history of infection-associated cancer because their existence was first recognized as elements of cancer-causing viruses.

Over 50 years after Rous described the sarcoma which bears his name, Huebner and Todaro introduced the term oncogene[79]. Their paper set out a theory that most or all cells of vertebrates contain integrated retroviral DNA, and that all cancers result from expression of these 'oncogenes'. The concept of integration of retroviral DNA is now well established; Weiss has suggested that as much as 8% of the human genome is accounted for by what he describes as *'fossil retroviral genomes'*[80]. Although the term oncogene was a new coinage, the concept of cancer-causing genes within viral genomes was not.

Initially it was thought that oncogenes were of viral origin, having evolved to allow the virus to bypass the mechanisms which normally control cell growth and division. Later it was recognized that the virus had acquired elements of the host genome thus becoming better fitted to succeed in the Darwinian arms-race[81] between the viral invader and the host's defence mechanisms. The discovery was entirely unexpected; it was reported in 1976 by Bishop and Varmus[82], who subsequently received the Nobel Prize for their crucial discovery. Such genes were termed cellular oncogenes or proto-oncogenes – these titles are both inappropriate as the genes are normal functional, indeed indispensable, elements of the genome. Their normal function is to promote cell growth and division in response to appropriate stimuli; malignant disease occurs when these genes are expressed aberrantly.

Viruses are predisposed to acquisition of host genes since they rely on host cell enzymes and organelles to replicate and to produce new infective viral particles. Retroviruses use reverse transcriptase to produce a DNA copy of their genome and insinuate this genome within the host genome. Transcription of the embedded viral genome will direct the production of components of the viral particle and their assembly into a complete virion. During this process, it is unsurprising that at times elements of host genome become embedded in the viral genome. This is probably a relatively common event but in many cases the acquired host genetic material will harm the virus in some way and prevent replication; when the virus remains viable even though host genes are embedded, this will usually be innocuous to the host. It has been estimated that only around 50 of the 30 000 or so genes in human cells are capable of acting as oncogenes.

Strikingly, this is not a one-way process; as cited, Weiss has estimated that as much as 8% of the human genome is litter left behind by trespassing viruses. Most of this litter is harmless, by definition, since affected hosts have continued to contribute to the gene pool. Fragments of retroviral DNA embedded in the host genome are termed 'endogenous retroviruses', in humans they are termed HER[83]. Huebner and Todaro believed that all cancers resulted from (re-) activation of such HER segments and considered the action of the viral oncogene to be a *sine qua non* of tumour development. It is now clear that there is no single pathway of oncogenesis; in some cases viral oncogenes play a vital role, whilst in others they play little or no part. For the purposes of this work, stably integrated endogenous retroviruses are not deemed to be infectious causes of cancer.

In the early 1970s, as cellular oncogenes were first being described, Harald zur Hausen was beginning the series of studies which would demonstrate that HPV is the causal agent for cervical cancer[84]. Zur Hausen eventually received a shared Nobel Prize for his work in this field.

Modern models of the development of malignancy in response to infection are complex, yet in many cases the mechanisms are still incompletely understood. Chapter 2 will review some basic concepts of cancer biology and microbiology and explore the current understanding of pathways by which infections may induce or drive malignant transformation.

References

1. Rothschild, B.M., Witzke, B.J. & Hershkovitz, I. (1999) Metastatic cancer in the Jurassic. *Lancet*, **354**, 398.

2. Poinar, G. & Poinar, R. (2005) Fossil evidence of insect pathogens. *Journal of Invertebrate Pathology*, **89**, 243–250.

3. Schell, J. & Van Montagu, M. (1977) Transfer, maintenance, and expression of bacterial Ti-plasmid DNA in plant cells transformed with *A. tumefaciens*. *Brookhaven Symposia in Biology*, **29**, 36–49.

4. Levin, I. & Levine, M. (1920) Malignancy of the crown gall and its analogy to animal cancer. *Journal of Cancer Research*, **5**, 243–260.

5. Smith, E.F. & Townsend, C.O. (1907) A plant-tumor of bacterial origin. *Science*, **26**, 671–673.

6. Lawrence, J.E.P. (1935) Appendix A. In: *Stone Age Races of Kenya* (ed. L.S.B. Leakey), p. 139. Oxford University Press, London.

7. Stathopoulos, G. (1975) Letter: Kanam mandible's tumour. *Lancet*, **1**, 165.

8. Phelan, J., Weiner, M.J., Ricci, J.L., Plummer, T., Gauld, S., Potts, R. & Bromage, T.G. (2007) Diagnosis of the pathology of the Kanam mandible. *Oral Surgery, Oral Medicine, Oral Pathology, Oral Radiology and Endodontology*, **103**, e20.

9. Stathopoulos, G.P. (1986) Bone tumours in antiquity. In: *Palaeo-Oncology: The Antiquity of Cancer* (ed. S. Retwas), pp. 13–26. Farrand Press, London.

10. Newby, J.A. & Howard, C.V. (2006) Environmental influences in cancer aetiology. *Journal of Nutritional and Environmental Medicine*, **15** (2–3), 56–114.

11. Breasted, J.H. (1930) *The Edwin Smith Surgical Papyrus*. University of Chicago Press, Chicago, Illinois.

12. Adams, F. (1886) *The Genuine Works of Hippocrates*. W. Wood, New York.

13. Hajdu, S.I. (2004) Greco-Roman thought about cancer. *Cancer*, **100**, 2048–2051.

14. Reedy, J. (1975) Galen on cancer and related diseases. *Clio Medica*, **10**, 227–238.

15. Vesalius, A. (1543) De humani corporis fabrica (On the structure of the human body). University of Padua, Padua.

16. Ackernecht, E.H. (1958) Historical notes on cancer. *Medical History*, **2**, 114–119.

17. Hunton, A. (1587) Of the nature and divers kinds of cancers or cankers – translated from "De cancri natura et curatione" by Benoit Textor. Robert Waldergrave, London.

18. Deshaies-Gendron, C. (1701) Recherches sur la nature et la guerison des cancers (Studies on the nature and treatment of cancer). Laurent d'Houry, Paris.

19. McGrew, R.E. (1985) *Encyclopedia of Medical History*. Macmillan Press, London.

20. Beckett, W. (1712) New discoveries relating to the cure of cancers… in a letter to a friend to which is added; A solution of some curious problems by William Beckett, surgeon. George Strahan, London.

21. Martin, H., Ehrlich, H. & Butler, F. (1950) J. Marion Sims – pioneer cancer protagonist. *Cancer*, **3**, 189–204.

22. Virchow, R. (1858) Die Cellularpathologie in ihrer Begründung auf physiologische und patholo-gische Gewebelehre. A. Hirschwald, Berlin.

23. Triolo, V.A. (1969) The institution for investigating the nature and cure of cancer. A study of four excerpts. *Medical History*, **13**, 11–28.

24. Hodgkin, T. (1843) On the anatomical characters of some adventitious structures, being an attempt to point out the relation between the microscopic characters and those which are discernible by the naked eye. *Medico Chirurgical Transactions*, **26**, 242–285.

25. Javier, R.T. & Butel, J.S. (2008) The history of tumor virology. *Cancer Research*, **68**, 693–706.

26. Borrel, A. (1903) Epithélioses infectieuses et épithéliomas. *Annales de l'Institut Pasteur*, **17**, 81–122.

27. Rous, P. (1910) A transmissible avian neoplasm. (Sarcoma of the common fowl.) *The Journal of Experimental Medicine*, **12**, 696–705.

28. Rous, P. (1911) Transmission of a malignant new growth by means of a cell-free filtrate. *JAMA*, **56**, 198.

29. Ellerman, W. & Bang, O. (1908) Experimentelle Leukäemie bei Hühnern. *Zentralblatt für Bakteriologie, Parasitenkunde, Infektionskrankheiten und Hygiene*, **46**, 595–609.

30. Lockhart-Mummery, J.P. (1932) The origin of tumours. *BMJ*, **ii**, 121.

31. Milt, H. (1969) Viruses and cancer. *CA: A Cancer Journal for Clinicians*, **19**, 219–227.

32. Van Epps, H.L. (2005) Peyton Rous: Father of the tumor virus. *The Journal of Experimental Medicine*, **201**, 320.

33. Rous, P., Murphy, J.B. & Tytler, W.H. (1912) A filterable agent the cause of a second chicken-tumor, an osteochondroma. *JAMA*, **59**, 1793–1794.

34. Shope, R.E. (1932) A filterable virus causing tumor-like condition in rabbits and its relationship to virus myxomatosum. *The Journal of Experimental Medicine*, **56**, 803–822.

35. Shope, R.E. & Hurst, E.W. (1933) Infectious papillomatosis of rabbits with notes on histopathology. *The Journal of Experimental Medicine*, **58**, 607–624.

36. Fibiger, J. (1913) Recherches sur un nématode et sur sa faculté de provoquer des néformations papillomateuses et carcinomateuses dans l' estomac du rat. Académie Royale Des Sciences et Des Lettres De Danemark.

37. Fibiger, J. (1918) Investigations on the Spiroptera cancer, III: On the transmission of *Spiroptera neoplastica* (*Gongylonema neoplasticum*) to the rat as a means of producing cancer experimentally. *Kongelige Danske Videnskabernes Selskab Biologistic Meddelelser*, **1**, 9.

38. Passey, R.D., Leese, A. & Knox, J.C. (1935) Spiroptera cancer and dietary deficiency. *Journal of Pathology and Bacteriology*, **40**, 198–205.

39. Raju, T.N. (1998) The Nobel chronicles. 1926: Johannes Andreas Grib Fibiger (1867–1928). *Lancet*, **352**, 1635.

40. Cramer, W. (1937) Papillomatosis in the forestomach of the rat and its bearing on the work of Fibiger. *American Journal of Cancer*, **31**, 537–555.

41. Fibiger, J. (1927) Investigations on *Spiroptera carcinoma* and the experimental induction of cancer – Nobel lecture. In: *Les Prix Nobel en 1926*, pp. 122–150. Imprimaterie Royale P. A. Norstedt & Somer, Stockholm.

42. Vogt, P.K. (1996) Peyton Rous: Homage and appraisal. *FASEB Journal*, **10**, 1559–1562.

43. Rous, P. (1967) The challenge to man of the neoplastic cell – Nobel lecture. In: *Les Prix Nobel en 1966*, pp. 162–171. Imprimaterie Royale P. A. Norstedt & Soner, Stockholm.

44. Kendall, S.D., Linardie, C.M., Adam, S.J. & Counter, C.M. (2005) A network of genetic events sufficient to convert normal human cells to a tumorigenic state. *Cancer Research*, **65**, 9824–9828.

45. Roscoe, B. Jackson Memorial Laboratory Staff (1933) The existence of non-chromosomal influence in the incidence of mammary tumors in mice. *Science*, **78**, 465–466.

46. Bittner, J. (1936) Some possible effects of nursing on the mammary gland tumor incidence in mice. *Science*, **84**, 162.

47. Bryan, W.R., Kahler, H., Shimkin, M.B. & Andervont, H.B. (1942) Extraction and ultracentrifugation of mammary tumor inciter of mice. *Journal of the National Cancer Institute*, **2**, 451–455.

48. Coffin, J.M., Hughes, S.H. & Varmus, H.E. (1997) A brief chronicle of retrovirology. In: *Retroviruses at the National Center for Biotechnology Information* (eds J.M. Coffin, S.H. Hughes & H.E. Varmus). NCBI, Bethesda, Maryland.

49. Shah, K.V., Bang, F.B. & Abbey, H. (1972) Considerations for epidemiologic studies to test the hypothesis of viral causation of human breast cancer. *Journal of the National Cancer Institute*, **48**, 1035–1038.

50. Lawson, J.S., Tran, D. & Rawlinson, W.D. (2001) From Bittner to Barr: A viral, diet and hormone breast cancer aetiology hypothesis. *Breast Cancer Research*, **3**, 81–85.

51. Burkitt, D.P. (1958) A sarcoma involving the jaws of African children. *British Journal of Surgery*, **46**, 218–223.

52. Burkitt, D.P. & O'Conor, G.T. (1961) Malignant lymphoma in African children. 1. A clinical syndrome. *Cancer*, **14**, 258–269.

53. O'Conor, G.T. (1961) Malignant lymphoma in African children. II. A pathological entity. *Cancer*, **14**, 270–283.

54. Coakley, D. (2006) Denis Burkitt and his contribution to haematology/oncology. *British Journal of Haematology*, **135**, 17–25.

55. Burkitt, D.P. (1962) A tumour safari in east and central Africa. *British Journal of Cancer*, **16**, 379–386.

56. Epstein, M.A., Achong, B.G. & Barr, Y.M. (1964) Virus particles in cultured lymphoblasts from Burkitt's lymphoma. *Lancet*, **1**, 702–703.

57. Epstein, M.A. (2001) Historical background. *Philosophical Transactions of the Royal Society of London B: Biological Sciences*, **356**, 413–420.

58. Baer, R. et al. (1984) DNA sequence and expression of the B95-8 Epstein–Barr virus genome. *Nature*, **310**, 207–211.

59. de-The, G., Day, N.E. et al. (1978) Epidemiological evidence for causal relationship between Epstein–Barr virus and Burkitt's lymphoma from Ugandan prospective study. *Nature*, **274**, 756–761.

60. IARC (1997) Epstein–Barr virus. *IARC Monographs on the Evaluation of Carcinogenic Risk to Humans*, **70**, 47. IARC Press, Lyon.

61. Centers for Disease Control and Prevention (1985) Revision of the case definition of acquired immunodeficiency syndrome for national reporting – United States. *Morbidity and Mortality Weekly Report*, **34**, 373–375.

62. Chêne, A., Donati, D., Guerreiro, A.O., Levitsky, V., Chen, O., Falk, K.I., Orem, J., Kironde, F., Wahlgren, M. & Bejerano, M.T. (2007) A molecular link between malaria and Epstein–Barr virus reactivation. *PLoS Pathogens*, **3**, 1–9.

63. van den Bosch, C. (2004) Is endemic Burkitt's lymphoma an alliance between three infections and a tumour promoter? *Lancet Oncology*, **5**, 738–746.

64. Ferry, J.A. (2006) Burkitt's lymphoma: Clinicopathological features and differential diagnosis. *Oncologist*, **11**, 375–383.

65. Atwood, K.C. (November 2004) Bacteria, ulcers and ostracism? *Skeptical Enquirer*, **26** (6).

66. Bizzozero, G. (1892) Sulle ghiandole tubulari del tube gastroenterico e sui rapporti dell'ero coll epithelo de rivestimento della mucosa. *Atti Della Reale Academia Delle Scienze Di Torino*, **28**, 233–251.

67. Warren, J.R. (1983) Unidentified curved bacilli on gastric epithelium in active chronic gastritis. *Lancet*, 1273–1275.

68. Warren, J.R. (2006) Helicobacter: The ease and difficulty of a new discovery (Nobel lecture). *ChemMedChem*, **1**, 672–685.

69. Koch, R. (1882) Die Aetiologie der tuberkulose. *Berliner Klinischen Wochenschrift*, **15**, 221–230.

70. Marshall, B.J., Armstrong, J.A., McGechie, D.B. & Glancy, R.J. (1985) Attempt to fulfill Koch's postulates for pyloric Campylobacter. *The Medical Journal of Australia*, **142**, 436–439.

71. Marshall, B. (2006) Helicobacter connections. *ChemMedChem*, **1**, 783–802.

72. Fossmark, R., Qvigstad, G. & Waldum, H.L. (2008) Gastric cancer: Animal studies on the risk of hypoacidity and hypergastrinemia. *World Journal of Gastroenterology*, **14**, 1646–1651.

73. IARC (1994) Schistosomes, liver flukes and *Helicobacter pylori*. *IARC Monographs on the Evaluation of Carcinogenic Risk to Humans*, **61**, 177.

74. Heidland, A., Klassen, A., Rutkowski, P. & Bahner, U. (2006) The contribution of Rudolf Virchow to the concept of inflammation: What is still of importance? *Journal of Nephrology*, 19(Suppl. 10), S102–S109.

75. Akhter, Y., Ahmed, I., Devi, S.M. & Ahmed, N. (2007) The co-evolved *Helicobacter pylori* and gastric cancer: Trinity of bacterial virulence, host susceptibility and lifestyle. *Infectious Agents and Cancer*, **2**, 2.

76. Watson, J.D. & Crick, F.H.C. (1953) Molecular structure of nucleic acids: A structure for deoxyribose nucleic acid. *Nature*, **171**, 737–738.

77. Crick, F.H.C. (1970) Central dogma of molecular biology. *Nature*, **227**, 561–563.

78. Crawford, L.V. & Crawford, E.M. (1961) The properties of Rous sarcoma virus purified by density gradient centrifugation. *Virology*, **13**, 227–232.

79. Huebner, R.J. & Todaro, G.J. (1969) Oncogenes of RNA tumor viruses as determinants of cancer. *Proceedings of the National Academy of Sciences of the United States of America*, **64**, 1087–1094.

80. Weiss, R.A. (2006) The discovery of endogenous retroviruses. *Retrovirology*, **3**, 67.

81. Dawkins, R. & Krebs, J.R. (1979) Arms races between and within species. *Proceedings of the Royal Society of London B*, **205**, 489–511.

82. Stéhelin, D., Varmus, H.E., Bishop, J.M. & Vogt, P.K. (1976) DNA related to the transforming gene(s) of avian sarcoma viruses is present in normal avian DNA. *Nature*, **260**, 170–173.

83. Kurth, R. & Bannert, N. (2010) Beneficial and detrimental effects of human endogenous retroviruses. *International Journal of Cancer*, **126**, 306–314.

84. zur Hausen, H., Meinhof, W., Scheiber, W. & Bornkamm, G.W. (1974) Attempts to detect virus-specific DNA sequences in human tumors: I. Nucleic acid hybridizations with complementary RNA of human wart virus. *International Journal of Cancer*, 13, 650–656.

2 The global burden

It has been estimated that infection-associated cancers (IACs) make up slightly more than one-quarter of the cancer burden in the developing world – and almost 18% of the global burden. There is a very uneven distribution of this burden. A greater incidence of cases is seen in the developing world and, within the developed world, members of poorer socio-economic strata tend to show higher rates.

Epidemiology of infection-associated cancer

Epidemiology is customarily divided into two arms – descriptive and analytical; the former treats numbers of cases, while the latter is concerned with studying the causes of disease. The scale of IAC differs between the economically advanced nations – the developed world – and the less advanced nations – the developing world. This difference can largely be explained by differing age profiles and standards of hygiene, but there are also significant variations in incidence within communities with comparable socio-economic backgrounds. It is clear that for many, probably all, IAC there are important cofactors which influence the probability of a person with the infection developing cancer. Commonly, the infection is a necessary, but not sufficient, risk factor for the associated cancer. Descriptive epidemiology detects the differing incidences of disease in different communities; analytical epidemiology seeks to explain those differences. There are wide geographical variations in the incidence of IACs[1] (see Table 2.1).

The magnitude of the differences in Table 2.1 depends on the interactions between several factors:

- Differing incidence of relevant infections
- Timing of infection
- Variability in the biology of the infectious agent(s)

Infectious Causes of Cancer, first edition. By Ken Campbell. Published 2011 by John Wiley & Sons Ltd.
© 2011 John Wiley & Sons Ltd.

Table 2.1 Geographical variation in incidence rates of IACs.

Site	High Population	Rate	Low Population	Rate	Ratio H/L
Nasopharynx					
Male	Hong Kong	28.5	Ecuador, Quito	0.1	285
Female	Hong Kong	11.2	UK – Birmingham, regions of Scotland	0.1	112
Stomach					
Male	Japan, Yamagata	93.3	India, Ahmedabad	2.1	44.4
Female	Japan, Yamagata	42.9	India, Ahmedabad The Gambia	1.5	28.6
Liver					
Male	Thailand, Khon Kaen China, Qidong	90.0	The Netherlands, Maastricht	0.8	112.5
Female	Thailand, Khon Kaen	38.3	Canada, Prince Edward Island	0.1	383
Hodgkin lymphoma					
Male	Italy, Parma	4.5	China, Qidong Japan, Yamagata	0.1	45
Female	US, Hawaii: Chinese	5.0	Japan, Hiroshima The Gambia	0.1	50
Cervix uteri	Peru, Trujillo	54.6	Israel: non-Jews	2.6	21

Note: Age standardized rates per 100 000.

■ Genetic variation in host susceptibility
  o To infection
  o To malignant complications of infection
■ Incidence of cofactors, e.g. smoking, aflatoxin exposure

This is not merely a consequence of variability in susceptibility to cancer of any type between populations; the incidence of liver cancer in the male population of Qidong district in China is one of the highest in the world, whereas the same population has one of the lowest rates of Hodgkin lymphoma. It is possible that genetic differences between populations may account for at least a proportion of the variance in incidence[2].

Epidemiology of infections and associated cancers

Epstein–Barr virus

In all communities that have been studied, Epstein–Barr virus (EBV) has been found to be ubiquitous, with almost all adults showing serological evidence of past infection. Over 90% of all adults have persistent, usually lifelong, latent EBV

Table 2.2 Causal contribution of EBV infection to various human cancers.

Malignancy	Subtype	EBV-positive (%)
Burkitt's lymphoma	Endemic	>95
	Non-endemic	15–30
Hodgkin lymphoma	Mixed cellularity	70
	Lymphocyte-depleted	>95
	Nodular sclerosing	10–40
	Lymphocyte-predominant	<5
Non-Hodgkin lymphoma	Nasal T/natural killer (NK)	>90
	Angioimmunoblastic lymphadenoplasty	Unknown
Nasopharyngeal carcinoma	Anaplastic	>95
Breast cancer	Medullary carcinoma Adenocarcinoma	0–50
Gastric cancer	Lymphoepithelioma-like	>90
	Adenocarcinoma	5–25
Post-transplant lymphoproliferative disorder (PTLD)		>90
AIDS-associated lymphoma	Immunoblastic primary central nervous system lymphoma (IP-CNS)	>95
	Other	30–50
Leiomyosarcoma in immunosuppressed patients		Frequent

infection – a latent infection is one in which the virus is present living within host cells without lysing those cells and without causing disease[3]. Early infection involves cells within the nasopharynx, while latent, lifelong infection is of memory B lymphocytes. In the developing world infection occurs in early childhood with no clinical evidence of infection. In the developed world infection occurs later, possibly with a young person's first kiss – this may cause glandular fever (infectious mononucleosis, IM) known colloquially as 'kissing disease'[4].

The first form of cancer to be definitely linked with an infectious agent was endemic Burkitt's lymphoma (BL) – the commonest malignancy in malarial areas of sub-Saharan Africa. Three clinical variants of BL are recognized[5]:

(1) Endemic (African) – nearly all cases are EBV positive
(2) Sporadic – 15–30% of cases are EBV positive
(3) Immunodeficiency-related
    (a) HIV/AIDS – almost all cases are EBV positive
    (b) Solid organ transplant recipients – commonly but not uniformly EBV positive

EBV is a contributory factor in a number of other human cancers. Table 2.2 summarizes the current view on the causal contribution of EBV to human cancers.

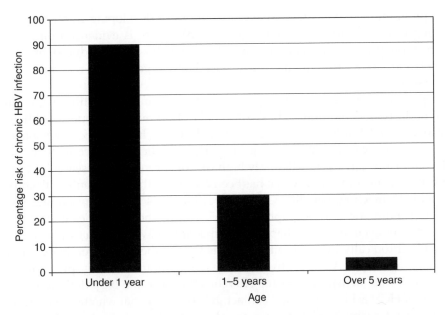

Figure 2.1 Percentage probability of chronic HBV infection by age of exposure. (Data from Mast *et al.*[9,10].)

EBV-associated nasopharyngeal cancer (EANPC) has a geographical distribution centred on regions of China and South-East Asia. This appears to be primarily associated with genetic factors, as incidence is high in Cantonese males wherever they live, but widespread consumption of salted fish is a cofactor[6].

Hepatitis viruses

Hepatitis B (HBV) is an extremely common virus; the *World Cancer Report* states that '*Approximately two billion people are infected worldwide, and more than 400 million are chronic (lifelong) carriers of HBV*'[7]. Hepatitis B infection is the principal causal factor in hepatocellular carcinoma (HCC) which represents about 80% of all cases of liver cancer; over half of the worldwide incidence of HCC is attributable to chronic HBV infection[8]. Chronic carrier status occurs most frequently when an individual is infected early in life and is associated with a significantly higher risk of developing cirrhosis and liver cancer; infection in adult life usually causes acute, symptomatic infection and resolves rapidly (see Figure 2.1).

Early infection is most common in the developing world, a fact which is reflected in the geographical distribution of chronic hepatitis B infection[10]. Globally, hepatitis B infection causes more deaths than any other carcinogen except tobacco smoke; it is estimated that, in total, hepatitis B causes around 1.2 million deaths annually[11]. The principal mode of transmission of HBV in the developing world and in deprived socio-economic groups is perinatal and this can be effectively blocked by a programme of neonatal vaccination; the risk of developing chronic hepatitis leading to HCC is low for adult-acquired HBV. There is evidence from the US vaccination programme that the impact can be drastically reduced by infant inoculation[12]; other programmes have selectively targeted high-risk adults with some success[13].

Hepatitis C virus (HCV), although less common than HBV, is still a major cause of morbidity and mortality. HCV infects about 80 million people worldwide[7]; unlike HBV, HCV infection during adult life leads to chronic infection in a majority (75–85%) of cases[14]. Epidemiological evidence indicates that co-infection with HBV and HCV carries a particularly high risk of chronic liver disease, leading to cirrhosis and eventually HCC[12]; it has been estimated that in patients with chronic hepatitis B infection, hepatitis C superinfection rates range from around 9% to 13% depending on the geographic region[15]. One of the difficulties in estimating rates of co-infection is that hepatitis B infection may be 'serologically silent' in patients chronically infected with hepatitis C[16]. As there is currently no vaccine available against HCV, preventive measures centre upon blocking spread of infection – this may be easier than for HBV or HIV since the only definite route of spread of HCV is blood to blood contact. It is controversial whether heterosexual contact can transmit the infection in the absence of bleeding[17]; anal intercourse is likely to carry a relatively high risk of blood–blood contact. It is accepted that if heterosexual transmission does occur it is much less common than for HBV or HIV. In the developed world an epidemic of HCV infection was seen to coincide with increased use of blood transfusion and parenteral therapies[18] – screening of donors and improvement of healthcare conditions has virtually eliminated this mode of spread in the developed world, although it is still a significant problem in poorer countries.

HCV has also been implicated in other forms of cancer, particularly certain subtypes of non-Hodgkin lymphoma (NHL)[19] and Hodgkin lymphoma[20].

Delta virus (hepatitis D virus, HDV) is an incomplete hepatitis virus which is dependent on co-infection with HBV for transcription and replication[21]; there is evidence that HCV patients who are co-infected with HBV and HDV develop HCC at a younger age than mono-infected patients[22]. The International Agency for Research on Cancer (IARC) considers HDV to be 'unclassifiable' as regards carcinogenic potential[23]. Hepatitis G is a more recently identified hepatitis virus, thought to be related to hepatitis C – its epidemiology and potential carcinogenicity are not yet clearly defined[24].

Human papillomaviruses

There are over 100 variants of papillomaviruses which infect humans; of these around 40 types typically infect mucosal epithelium. Strains are classified as high- or low-risk on the basis of the oncogenic potential of the strain; low-risk strains may cause benign lesions such as warts. HPV 16 and 18 are the commonest high-risk strains; HPV 6 and 11 are the commonest low-risk strains causing benign neoplasms. The majority of papillomavirus infections cause only silent infection or benign lesions, including common warts and genital warts. A small number of high-risk strains account for about 70% of cervical cancer incidence; high-risk strains are also implicated as causes of head and neck cancer, skin cancer, penile cancer and oral cancer. Low-risk strains are associated with benign tumours such as skin warts and genital warts. Classification of papillomavirus is on the basis of differences in the DNA sequence within three viral gene regions: E6, E7 and L1[25].

Cervical infection

It is extremely difficult to determine the extent of HPV infection in women because almost all infections are cleared within 2 years[26]. HPV is certainly the most prevalent sexually transmitted infection in the world, with about 70–80% of sexually active people being infected at some time in their life[27], and is the only carcinogen so far accepted as being a necessary causal agent for development of any cancer[28]. Worldwide, a study showed that 99.7% of cases of cervical cancer contained HPV DNA[29]; the other 0.3% are most probably false negatives, although the possibility of non-HPV-associated cases cannot be excluded. Cervical cancer is the second most common gynaecological cancer in the world[30] after breast cancer. In many areas of the developing world, cervical cancer is *the* most common form; where facilities for screening are limited, cervical cancer is often the leading cause of cancer death in women. Indeed this was the case in the US as late as the 1930s[31].

Other sites

In addition to male and female genitalia, there are other sites which commonly harbour HPV; for each of these sites there is evidence that HPV is capable of acting as a carcinogen. The same strains that cause cervical cancer may be found in other anogenital sites in both men and women. The low-risk strains 6 and 11 are the most frequent causes of genital warts, which usually resolve spontaneously and very rarely progress to high-grade dysplasia and almost never to invasive cancer[32]. High-risk strains 16 and 18 are the most frequent HPV strains causally associated with cervical cancer; type 16 may also cause other anogenital cancers in men and women[33].

It is probable that skin infection with papillomavirus is ubiquitous – 'probably everybody is infected over long periods, if not throughout life, with these viruses'[34]. HPV-associated squamous-cell skin cancer appears to be principally a condition encountered in immunosuppressed individuals[35]. Papillomaviruses are strongly implicated as the causes of a subset of head and neck cancer[36]; the strongest risk factors for this site are alcohol consumption and tobacco use, but increasingly patients are being seen who lack these classic risk factors. HPV 16 may appear to play a significant causal role in this subgroup of cases; the site of tumour differs with apparent cause – smoking is most strongly associated with laryngeal cancer, alcohol with oral cancer and HPV 16 with pharyngeal cancer[37]. The most likely route of transmission is oral sex[38], although mouth to mouth contact cannot be excluded[36].

The importance of the discovery of the relationship between HPV infection and cervical cancer is indicated by the Nobel Prize for Physiology or Medicine awarded to Harold zur Hauser in 2008 (shared with Luc Montagnier and Barre-Sinoussi, who discovered HIV)[39].

Human T lymphotropic virus-1

Human T lymphotropic virus-1 (HTLV-1) is also referred to as human T-cell leukaemia virus-1, but the 'lymphotropic' form will be used throughout this book. HTLV-1 is the causal agent for a lymphoid malignancy (adult T-cell leukaemia/lymphoma, ATLL) first described in 1977[40]. It was found in 16 adults with T-cell leukaemia; the authors noted that most cases originated from a specific area within Japan. The final sentence of their paper reads, 'Genetic background may play an important role but other factors such as oncogenic virus infections must be explored'.

In 1980, a novel retrovirus was isolated from malignant T-cells[41], and by 1982 this had been found in cells from most cases of ATLL[42]. The presence of the HTLV-1 virus is now part of the case definition of ATLL, although 100% of patients with ATLL are HTLV-1 positive, only a very small percentage of those infected with HTLV-1 develop any associated disease. In Japan, it has been reported that the cumulative incidence rate of ATLL in HTLV-1 carriers is 4.5% in males and 2.6% in females[43]. Given that there are estimated to be 15–20 million HTLV-1 carriers worldwide[44], even this low rate translates to a large number of individuals at risk of developing cancer. Although there have been reports speculating on a link with other cancers, a recent review cites ATLL as the only associated malignant disease[45].

Human herpesvirus 8/Kaposi sarcoma herpesvirus

Kaposi sarcoma-associated herpesvirus (KSHV) is the causal agent of Kaposi sarcoma (KS) and of primary effusion lymphoma (PEL)[46]. The virus has a limited geographic distribution compared with other human herpesviruses (HHV), which are ubiquitous; human herpesvirus 8 (HHV-8) infection rates are low in the US and most European countries (<3%), intermediate in Mediterranean regions (up to 25%) and high in central African countries (>50%)[47]. HHV-8-linked malignancies are seen almost exclusively in immunosuppressed individuals, who can be grouped into four categories (Table 2.3).

The first three categories in Table 2.3 were encountered in at-risk populations prior to the emergence of the AIDS global pandemic. Epidemic KS was not known pre-AIDS.

Classic
KS was first described in 1872[48,49] as a small series of cases in men over the age of 40, all of them being Western European. The typical classic Kaposi sarcoma (CKS) patient is an elderly Ashkenazi Jewish male of Mediterranean or Eastern European descent[50]; Israel has one of the highest incidences in the world of CKS, reflecting the

Table 2.3 Clinical settings in which Kaposi sarcoma may be encountered.

	Population	Ages	Known cofactors
Classic	Mediterranean and Ashkenazi Jewish	Over 60	
Endemic	Equatorial Africa children and older males	Children	Podoconiosis? Iron absorbed from soil
Iatrogenic	Immunosuppressed patients, especially post-transplant	All ages	Immunosuppressive therapy and/or illness
Epidemic	Mainly homo- and bisexual HIV infected men	Younger males	HIV immunosuppression; exposure to semen? Poppers?

ethnic origin of many Israeli citizens[51]. This form now accounts for a very small percentage of cases in comparison with the epidemic (HIV-related) form described below. Other than age, no particular cofactors have been described as influencing the risk of CKS. Typically, lesions are confined to the skin and subcutaneous tissues of the lower limbs, which means CKS does not significantly shorten lifespan[52].

Endemic (African)
KS is seen in an endemic form in parts of Africa, with geographical and anatomical distributions which both strikingly resembled that of a form of elephantiasis called podoconiosis[53]. Podoconiosis is an endemic non-filarial elephantiasis seen in populations who live at high elevations in areas with heavy rainfall and volcanic soils and who habitually go barefoot on those soils[54]. Irritant particles from the soil penetrate bare skin and eventually become lodged in, and block the lymphatic vasculature[55]. The iron content of the soil particles may cause localized immunoparesis in the lower extremities, which matches the distribution of lesions in endemic African KS[56]. Although endemic KS occurs in regions of Africa where podoconiosis is not common[57], podoconiosis may be causal where the two conditions do coexist. It would be extremely uncommon for a patient with this form of KS to present in a European or North American healthcare setting.

Iatrogenic
Patients therapeutically immunosuppressed post organ transplantation have a much higher incidence of KS than the populations from which they are drawn. KS occurs in about 0.4–0.6% of recipients of solid organs – about 150–200 times commoner than in the general population[58]. A comparison between renal transplant recipients and a control population of the same ethnic origin showed a 400–500-fold increase in KS incidence in the former[59]; this may be a more accurate indication of the increased risk of KS. Mendez stated in 2000 that KS made up more than 5% of all new tumours seen in the transplant recipient population, and that the incidence in that population was rising[60].

Epidemic

In 1981, reports were published of KS occurring in previously unaffected populations – young homosexual males; this is known to have been the first evidence of
the AIDS pandemic. KS was the first malignancy to be linked to HIV infection; it is
now one of several AIDS-defining malignancies. HIV infection is not synonymous
with AIDS; AIDS is defined as opportunistic infection or certain defined malignancies in an HIV-positive individual.

KS is sometimes seen in gay men with high-risk behaviour who are HIV negative. It has been suggested that this may be caused by chronic immunosuppression
induced by high semen load and/or use of recreational drugs such as amyl nitrite
(poppers). Further evidence for additional risk factors beyond HIV positivity is
the observation that KS is seen in 21–40% of men having sex with men in contrast
to only 1.6% of children with AIDS and 1% of haemophiliacs who have AIDS[52]. The
incidence of KS in the HIV-positive population has shown a marked decline in
developed countries, where highly active antiretroviral therapy (HAART) is
widely available[61], suggesting that other cofactors affecting the risk of gay males
have little impact in the absence of HIV.

Other viruses

Simian virus 40

A number of other viruses have been cited as possible causes of malignancy, but in
each case the evidence is incomplete and/or unpersuasive. One of the longest-
standing debates is whether simian virus 40 (SV 40), a virus which contaminated
batches of polio-vaccine, has caused cancers in those who were exposed. This has
yet to be declared a carcinogen by the IARC, which is normally considered the
definitive criterion. Perhaps the strongest evidence relates to mesothelioma, in
which SV 40 is believed to act as a co-carcinogen with asbestos, but even here the
IARC states that *'Whether a latent SV 40 infection is a causal factor in the development
of mesothelioma, remains to be assessed'*[62].

SV 40 has been demonstrated to be carcinogenic both in vitro and in vivo in
various animal species[63]. In an in vitro study of the minimal set of genetic changes
required to trigger malignant transformation, one of the four changes was insertion of the large T antigen of SV 40, which binds to and inhibits both the retinoblastoma (Rb) tumour suppressor and p53, which is often known as the 'guardian of
the genome'[64]. The strongest epidemiological evidence, as stated, is probably that
for mesothelioma; even here one can find in papers published in the same year the
contradictory assertions that *'no association between SV 40 prevalence and asbestos-
corrected male pleural cancer can be demonstrated'*[65] and that *'mineral fibers and viruses
can be cocarcinogens and suggest that lower amounts of asbestos may be sufficient to cause
MM in individuals infected with SV 40'*[63]. Pending further evidence the most that can
be said is that SV 40 is unlikely to contribute other than minimally to IAC, either
in the UK or globally. Given the central role of asbestos exposure in mesothelioma

carcinogenesis and the time lag between asbestos exposure and mesothelioma, Peto has predicted that mesothelioma deaths in Britain will peak around 2020 and then decline very rapidly[66].

Merkel cell polyomavirus[67],[68]

In 2008, a novel polyomavirus was isolated from cells of Merkel cell carcinoma (MCC), a rare neuroendocrine skin cancer[69]. The organism was discovered by the same husband and wife team which isolated HHV-8 from KS samples[70]. Preliminary studies strongly suggest a causal link between Merkel cell polyomavirus (MCP) and MCC[71], although further studies will be required to confirm this; there is currently no IARC evaluation of Merkel cell virus (MCV).

Non-viral infections

Helicobacter pylori

The first humans to emerge from Africa carried *Helicobacter pylori* in their stomachs[72]; sequence similarity between *Helicobacter* species seen in humans and big cats suggests that the association goes back far further than this, and that ancestors of modern humans may have been carrying *H. pylori* 200 000 years ago[73]. Modern data indicates that around half of the world's population is infected with *H. pylori*[74], probably in early childhood in most cases[75]. This widely cited figure conceals great variation between populations and within populations; *H. pylori* infection is most prevalent in lower socio-economic groups and in families where parents or older siblings are already infected[76]. It has been estimated globally that differential rates of infection by social class may account for 50 000 cases per year of stomach cancer – about 8% of the total[77]. There is a striking difference between the age profile of incidence of infection in the developed and developing worlds[78].

In North America and Western Europe, there has been a significant, continuing decline in reported rates of infection[79,80]. Fewer than one in ten US children is found to be carrying *H. pylori* – an organism which was once present in almost every adult stomach[81]. Childhood infection rates reliably predict eventual adult rates; it has been shown that following eradication of *H. pylori* reinfection rates in adults are very low at ~0.4% per year[82]. The decline in incidence is probably multifactorial, relating to changes in demographics, community hygiene and antibiotic use[81]. As the rate of infection in the juvenile population falls, it will inevitably mean less exposure of children to sources of infection, implying even lower rates in succeeding generations.

H. pylori appears normally to be a harmless passenger in the stomach; a minority of patients develop dyspepsia and possibly a gastric ulcer, and an even smaller minority develop gastric cancer[83]. *H. pylori* infected individuals have an increased risk of non-cardia cancer, but lower risks of gastric cardia cancer and oesophageal cancer[84,85]. *H. pylori* infection is implicated in a high proportion of cases of gastric mucosa-associated lymphoid tissue (MALT) lymphomas[86]. Although few infected individuals develop cancer, the prevalence of *H. pylori* means that stomach cancer is the second most common cause of cancer-related death in the world[87]; almost two-thirds of gastric cancer incidence and mortality occurs in the developing world[88].

Schistosoma species

Schistosomes are multicellular parasites (trematodes, blood flukes) for which the definitive hosts are mammals including man; their intermediate hosts are freshwater snails. Any given species of schistosome has a restricted range of definitive hosts and a specific intermediate host; this in turn limits the geographic distribution[89,90].

In endemic areas the larval stage (cercaria) is found in stagnant fresh water – humans become infected when these penetrate the skin; they then migrate in the bloodstream to the liver. In the liver they mature into adults, which pair off and migrate to and lodge in tissue blood vessels. Adults of *Schistosoma japonicum* and *S. mansoni* lodge in the mesenteric veins; those of *S. haematobium* lodge in terminal venules in the wall of the bladder and genitourinary system. They release eggs which lodge in tissues or are excreted in either urine or faeces (depending on the species); when eggs enter water intermediate-stage larvae called miracidia hatch, invade water snails and continue the life cycle. When eggs lodge in tissues, which may include the urinary bladder, bower wall, liver, lung or other sites, they provoke a brisk immune response which appears necessary for maturation and release of eggs[91]. Chronic *S. haematobium* infection is recognized by the IARC as a class I carcinogen for bladder cancer[92]; the mechanism is incompletely understood but involves prolonged low-level inflammation – there is evidence that schistosome eggs from all species secrete immunomodulatory cytokines. Schistosomiasis may reduce the risk of autoimmune diseases, probably via such immunomodulation[93].

Schistosome species have complex life cycles, which can be summarized as:

- In the definitive host, cercariae develop into immature worms, pair off and lodge in blood vessels.
- Mature worms release eggs, which migrate to specific tissues or enter the environment in urine or faeces.
- In fresh water, eggs hatch, releasing miracidia, which penetrate an intermediate host – a freshwater snail.
- In the intermediate host, miracidia form sporocysts, which release free-swimming cercariae.
- Cercariae penetrate the skin of a definitive, mammalian, host and migrate via the circulation to the liver, where they lodge, and the cycle recommences.

Schistosomiasis cannot be transmitted outwith the endemic area as the intermediate hosts are absent and direct transmission between definitive hosts cannot occur. All cases of schistosomiasis seen in temperate countries have been imported from

Table 2.4 Global variation in proportion of bladder cancer associated with
S. haematobium infection.

Area	*S. haematobium* prevalence (%)	Bladder cancer		
			Attributable cases	
		Cases – 1990	%	Number
Eastern Africa	29.2	5 519	54	3 000
Middle Africa	30.3	1 955	55	1 000
Northern Africa	11.3	12 663	31	3 900
Southern Africa	10.2	1 260	29	400
Western Africa	32.6	2 686	57	1 500
Western Asia	1.2	7 349	5	370
Africa + Western Asia		31 500	32	10 200
Developing countries		123 167	8	10 200
Developed countries		156 957	0	
World		280 124	3	10 200

tropical or subtropical countries. This can be used to exclude the diagnosis in any person who has never travelled to a country where schistosomiasis is endemic; this is in contrast to other diseases such as malaria, where there are well-documented cases of transmission within the UK to persons who have never travelled abroad[94].

'Approximately 200 million people are infected globally in 76 countries and about 600 million are exposed to infection in tropical and subtropical regions of Africa, Asia, South America and the Caribbean'[95]. This makes it the second most common human parasitic infection after malaria which is estimated to infect between 300 and 500 million people[96]. About 85% of all cases and almost all of the most severe cases occur in African countries[97]. Schistosomiasis (also known as bilharzia) has been present in Egypt for over 3000 years[98]. Endemic bilharzia is more likely to be chronic, whereas traveller's bilharzia is likely to be acute. This is important because it is chronic disease which is associated with bladder cancer. There are significant differences between schistosomiasis-related bladder cancer and non-bilharzial cases. In countries where schistosomiasis is endemic most cases of bladder cancer are squamous cell carcinoma. In the developed world over 90% of bladder cancers are transitional cell carcinoma and the most common risk factor is cigarette smoking, considered responsible for about two-thirds of male cancers of this type and about one-third of female cases. Pisani *et al.* have estimated (as of 1990) the contribution of schistosomiasis to bladder cancer incidence in different world regions based on rates of *S. haematobium* infection and an assumed fivefold increase in risk[99] (Table 2.4).

Although *Schistosoma* sp. have a tropical and subtropical distribution they are easily acquired by tourists and may also present in immigrants who are long settled in the UK. The London School of Hygiene and Tropical Medicine (LSHTM) reported a sharp increase in cases between 1987 and 1994[100,101]; from a peak in 1999 the Health Protection Agency (HPA) reports a decline in laboratory reports of schistosomiasis[102]. The initial rise in cases was attributed to increases in UK overseas tourism but no explanation has been suggested for the recent decline in reports. The most common species reported in the UK is *S. haematobium* and the most common place of infection is sub-Saharan Africa, particularly Malawi.

In 1996, around 240 000 UK residents travelled to areas in Africa where schistosomiasis is endemic[101]; Whitty *et al.* report that 18% of asymptomatic travellers who had been exposed to risk of schistosomiasis, and who were screened at LSHTM, were found to be infected. This may be significant as acute infection is readily treatable while chronic infection may lead, after several decades, to bladder cancer. Although bilharzial bladder cancer contributes a very small percentage to the bladder cancer burden in the UK, it should be borne in mind as a risk factor for older patients who have spent long periods in endemic areas, especially sub-Saharan Africa.

The typical natural history of bilharzia-associated bladder cancer is acquisition of *S. haematobium* infection in early childhood, followed by many years of release of eggs by adults. The eggs lodge in vessels of the urinary bladder, causing an intense immune response, often leading to granuloma formation. In the third decade of the host's life, bladder cancer may develop. In endemic areas where early childhood infection is common there is limited data as to whether adult-acquired infection can lead to bladder cancer. Sustained childhood-acquired infection, in which adult parasites may survive in the host for 30 years or more[101], appears to involve a balance of Th-1 and Th-2 immune responses; the host–parasite interaction in adult-acquired infection may be quite different.

A special category exists of patients who may have been exposed to schistosomiasis risk before effective therapy for the acute condition was available – ex-service personnel who have served in areas where schistosomiasis is endemic. Use of NHS facilities to replace closed military hospitals may bring healthcare workers in contact with Gurkha personnel, who may have been infected with *S. mansoni* or *S. japonicum*.

It has been suggested that infection with *S. mansoni* or *S. japonicum* may be risk factors for liver cancer, or for other specific cancers. The IARC states that *'A number of cases of liver cancer, colorectal cancer, giant follicular lymphoma and some other cancers have been reported in association with S. mansoni infection'*, while *'Mortality from liver cancer and prevalence of infection with S. japonicum have been found to be positively correlated in Japan but not consistently so in China'*[92]. The IARC summarized the evidence as follows:

- There is *inadequate evidence* in humans for the carcinogenicity of infection with *S. mansoni*.
- There is *limited evidence* in humans for the carcinogenicity of infection with *S. japonicum*.
- Infection with *S. mansoni* is *not classifiable as to its carcinogenicity to humans* (*Group 3*).
- Infection with *S. japonicum* is *possibly carcinogenic to humans* (*Group 2B*).

Given that Group 2B, which includes *S. japonicum*, also includes coffee, there will be no further discussion in this text of cancer risks associated with blood flukes other than *S. haematobium*.

Eradication schemes have been mounted using molluscicides to kill snails, which act as intermediate hosts. The chemicals used are toxic and the schemes are labour-intensive and expensive. A better solution would be the provision of good sanitation (preventing contamination of water by urine and excreta) and supplies of guaranteed clean water for drinking, cooking and washing. Education schemes have had very limited success; it is of little value to warn populations of the danger of certain behaviour if no alternatives to at-risk behaviour are available[90].

Liver flukes[103]

Three closely related food-borne trematode species, *Opisthorchis viverrini*, *O. felineus* and *Clonorchis sinensis*, may infect humans. These conditions have much more limited geographic distributions than schistosomiasis. This may be because, unlike schistosomiasis, liver flukes have a complex life cycle, with two intermediate hosts, and can only enter the body by being ingested, usually in uncooked fish. The geographical distribution reflects the areas where contaminated fish are present and dishes containing uncooked fish are dietary staples. The Khon Kaen region of northern Thailand has the world's highest rate of cholangiocarcinoma at 84.6 cases per 100 000, the next highest is 2.8 per 100 000 in the Osaka prefecture of Japan, while typical rates in industrialized countries are less than 1 per 100 000[104]. According to Parkin, in Khon Kaen 90% of all liver cancers are cholangiocarcinoma; in all other regions for which data is cited, HCC is more common.

The liver flukes have a complex lifestyle – as with blood flukes, mammals including humans are the definitive hosts but, unlike blood flukes, there are two intermediate hosts and the final host can only be infected by ingestion of metacercariae. In the case of *O. viverrini*, these are usually within the flesh or skin of freshwater fish, which are eaten raw. Once established in the final host the flukes lodge in the bile duct – in a minority of cases this may trigger cholangitis, cholecystitis and cholangiocarcinoma.

The IARC categorizes liver flukes as[92]:

■ Infection with *O. viverrini* is *definitely carcinogenic in humans* (*Group 1*)
■ Infection with *O. felineus* is *not classifiable as to its carcinogenicity to humans* (*Group 3*)
■ Infection with *C. sinensis* is *probably carcinogenic in humans* (*Group 2A*)

Although cholangiocarcinoma (bile duct cancer) is a rare sequel of infection, the extremely high rates of infection in some areas lead to a significant cancer burden. It is believed that dietary nitrosamines act with *O. viverrini* to increase the risk of cholangiocarcinoma[105]; nitrosamines are present in the same raw fish which carries the parasite, but are also formed in the gut, and the level of formation may be increased by liver fluke infestation[106]. Locally produced Thai cigarettes contain high levels of nitrosamines and may contribute to carcinogenesis[107].

It is estimated that around 600 million people are potentially at risk of infection with liver flukes[108]; around 9 million people are infected with *O. viverrini*, around 1.5 million people carry *O. felineus* and about 7 million people have *C. sinensis*. Although the evidence for carcinogenic potential of *C. sinensis* is weaker than for *O. viverrini*, it is considered by the IARC as probably a causal factor for cholangiocarcinoma[92].

As with schistosomiasis, intermediate vectors for liver flukes are only found in the endemic areas and transmission cannot occur without these vectors. Unlike schistosomiasis these infections are not easily acquired by tourists and so are extremely rare outside the endemic areas. The HPA makes no mention of liver fluke infection in the UK as travel-associated infections[102] or in migrant populations[109]. Cholangiocarcinoma is also very rare except where liver fluke infestation, ingestion of raw fish *and* high nitrosamine exposure coincide. This deadly triad creates the Khon Kaen 'hot spot' for cholangiocarcinoma.

An adventurous traveller might sample *koi-pla*, the northern Thailand staple meal prepared with raw fish and thus become infected with *O. viverrini*. Chronic infection with eventual risk of cholangiocarcinoma is unlikely to ensue as severe infections, which are most strongly associated with bile duct cancer, are usually symptomatic and readily cured. A report from Israel[110] describes infection from imported raw fish; fortunately, absence of intermediate hosts in temperate climes precludes onward transmission. In the Israeli case, the fish had been imported from an area in Siberia – *O. felineus* is endemic in Kazakhstan, Russian Federation, Siberia and Ukraine, with an estimated 12.5 million people at risk of infection[108]. Infection risk is particularly high in Khon Kaen because raw (contaminated) fish is a staple element of the local diet. Although there are no reports of UK-diagnosed liver fluke infection it is still a possible diagnosis in anyone who has spent time in a high-risk area; a US review identified cases in immigrants, 25% of whom had been in the US for at least 5 years[111].

Cholangiocarcinoma occurs in the absence of liver fluke infection. The incidence of the intrahepatic form of this tumour has been rising markedly in areas of low endemicity, including Western Europe and the US; intriguingly, this is accompanied by a drop in the incidence of extrahepatic cholangiocarcinoma[112]. Control of parasite infestation in endemic areas might lead to a dramatic reduction in mortality from cholangiocarcinoma; globally the incidence is very low and the aetiology is poorly understood, offering little or no scope for prevention.

Criteria in cancer aetiology

In 1882 Robert Koch, a German microbiologist, published criteria for whether a specific illness was caused by a specific infectious organism[113]; these have come to be known as Koch's postulates. They have been adapted over the years and are now given as follows:

■ The incriminated agent can be cultured from lesions of the disease.
■ The incriminated agent does not occur as a fortuitous and non-pathogenic contaminant in individuals who are healthy or have other diseases.
■ The agent can be grown in pure culture.
■ The agent reproduces the disease when introduced into an appropriate host.
■ The agent can be recultured from the diseased host.

There are difficulties in applying Koch's postulates to virus infections – this is particularly the case for virus-associated cancers[114]. In 1990 a set of criteria were published[115] which combine epidemiological and virological guidelines; these are known as the *Evans–Mueller* guidelines:

Epidemiological guidelines

(1) Geographic distribution of viral infection corresponds with that of the tumour, adjusting for the presence of known cofactors.
(2) Viral markers are higher in case subjects than in matched control subjects.
(3) Viral markers precede tumour development, with a higher incidence of tumours in persons with markers than those without.
(4) Tumour incidence is decreased by viral infection prevention.

Virological guidelines

(1) Virus can transform cells in vitro.
(2) Viral genome is present in tumour cells, but not in normal cells.
(3) Virus induces the tumour in an experimental animal.

In 2004, the Cancer Etiology Branch of the US National Cancer Institute hosted a workshop entitled 'Validation of a causal relationship: criteria to establish etiology', to consider the special problems encountered in assessing the significance of putative cancer-causing agents. A report based on that workshop[116] identified 12 key issues; a full discussion of those issues would be beyond the scope of this text, but a list of them is given below. Carbone's paper discusses the background to each of these questions:

(1) With regard to current criteria, how to identify human carcinogens and improve these criteria to reflect new advances in scientific knowledge and state-of-the-art techniques (transcriptional profiling, proteomics and so on)?
(2) Should the criteria be the same for different agents (viruses, chemicals, physical agents, promoting agents versus initiating DNA-damaging agents)?
(3) Should the criteria be the same for the elderly, children, different sexes and genetic background?
(4) How can we integrate our new knowledge of molecular biology/pathogenesis with previous criteria to establish cancer aetiology more accurately and more promptly?
(5) Knowing the genetic/epigenetic changes that take place in cancer, can this information help us to identify the carcinogens that caused those changes?

(6) What is the hierarchy of state-of-the-art approaches needed for confirmation criteria, and which bioassays are critical for decisions: epidemiology, animal testing, cell culture, genomics and so forth?

(7) If a given agent alters key cellular mechanisms required for carcinogenesis (including inactivation of Rb and p53, activation of ras and of telomerase, tumour invasion, angiogenesis and metastasis), should such an agent be considered a human carcinogen?

(8) What is the present value of using tissue culture and animal experiments to identify human carcinogens?

(9) Can we integrate genetic predisposition to cancer to identify the carcinogens that individuals with these genetic changes are most susceptible to?

(10) We are screening populations using new molecular approaches (proteomics, methylation changes and so forth) to identify high-risk individuals. Can we use this information to identify the causes (i.e. the carcinogenic substances) responsible for these molecular changes?

(11) What are the most important biases and confounders in these bioassays? What are the main problems in interpretation of data, especially if agents demonstrate threshold effects and not conventional linear-dose responses?

(12) Modern epidemiological studies often depend on genetic, biochemical or viral assays that had not been developed in the 1960s when Hill's criteria to identify carcinogens were developed. How can we incorporate this information to improve the accuracy of Hill's epidemiological criteria to identify human carcinogens?

The last of these discussion points, concerning the applicability of the Bradford Hill criteria for assessing causal relationships, offered a list of how modern technology might assist in applying these criteria:

- **Strength**. Measuring and quantitating with greater accuracy and precision, resulting in smaller studies producing larger relative risk estimates.
- **Consistency**. Improved techniques with reduced measurement error will contribute to greater consistency among studies and potentially decreased publication bias.
- **Plausibility and biological coherence**. Defining downstream pathways more accurately.
- **Analogy**. Comparing at a broader level the events found in new technologies and, potentially, discovering new analogies never before suspected. This may lead to an easier path for use of these technologies.
- **Specificity**. The new studies are unlikely to help in its assessment; that requires the verification of external models to be useful.
- **Temporal relationships**. Defining relationships through these new studies will enable a more accurate assessment of exposure onset, leading to a better definition of latency.
- **Dose–response relationships**. Lowering the threshold of detection through new technologies and therefore helping to expand the range of dose–response

relationships. This will lead to more accurate measurements of the exposure dose–risk relation.

■ **Experimental evidence**. Defining pathways earlier and more quickly. They then can be expanded to prospective human epidemiological trials for more rapid validation.

Defining causal relationships between infections and cancers is often difficult. Typically there is a long latency between infection and development of a malignancy and one or more cofactors are required. Even HPV, deemed a necessary cause for cervical cancer, is not a sufficient cause. In most cases only a very small percentage of people carrying a given infection will go on to develop an associated malignancy. In some cases, such as *O. viverrini* and cholangiocarcinoma, an infection is common but associated cofactors are rare and geographically limited. In a 2004 review[117] the specific issues relating to infectious causes of cancer are discussed in detail; interestingly, the authors of this paper cite polyomaviruses (SV 40, BK and JC) as causes of mesothelioma and brain tumours, yet the IARC has not classified any of these as carcinogenic. Perhaps this just goes to show how difficult it is to draw definitive conclusions! The conclusion of a recent review was that the 95% confidence limits for numbers of human viruses yet to be discovered are a minimum of 38 species and a maximum of 562; they estimate that between 10 and 40 new species will be discovered by 2020[118].

References

1. Harras, A., Edwards, B.K., Blot, W.J. & Gloecklet Ries, L.A. (eds) (1996) *Cancer: Rates and Risks.* National Cancer Institute, National Institutes of Health, Bethesda, Maryland.

2. Zeng, Z., Guan, L., An, P., Sun, S., O'Brien, S.J. & Winkler, C.A. (2008) A population-based study to investigate host genetic factors associated with hepatitis B infection and pathogenesis in the Chinese population. *BMC Infectious Diseases,* **8**, 1.

3. Crawford, D.H. (2001) Biology and disease associations of Epstein-Barr virus. *Philosophical Transactions of the Royal Society B: Biological Sciences,* **356**, 461–473.

4. Bornkamm, G.W., Behrends, U. & Mautner, J. (2006) The infectious kiss: Newly infected B cells deliver Epstein-Barr virus to epithelial cells. *Proceedings of the National Academy of Sciences USA,* **103**, 7201–7202.

5. Ferry, J.A. (2006) Burkitt's lymphoma: Clinicopathological features and differential diagnosis. *Oncologist,* **11**, 375–383.

6. Yu, M.C., Ho, J.H., Lai, S.H. & Henderson, B.E. (1986) Cantonese-style salted fish as a cause of nasopharyngeal carcinoma: Report of a case-control study in Hong Kong. *Cancer Research,* **46**, 956–961.

7. Boyle, P. & Levin, B. (eds) (2008) Chronic infections. In: *World Cancer Report 2008,* pp. 128–135. International Agency for Research on Cancer, Lyon.

8. Boyle, P. & Levin, B. (eds) (2008) Liver cancer. In: *World Cancer Report 2008,* pp. 350–357. International Agency for Research on Cancer, Lyon.

9. Mast, E.E., Margolis, H.S., Fiore, A.E., *et al.* (2005) A comprehensive immunization strategy to eliminate transmission of hepatitis B virus infection in the United States: Recommendations of the Advisory Committee on Immunization Practices (ACIP) Part 1: Immunization of infants, children, and adolescents. *MMWR Recommendations and Reports,* **54**, 1–31.

10. Mast, E.E., Weinbaum, C.M., Fiore, A.E., *et al.* (2006) A comprehensive immunization strategy to eliminate transmission of hepatitis B virus infection in the United States: Recommendations of the Advisory Committee on Immunization Practices (ACIP) Part II: Immunization of adults. *MMWR Recommendations and Reports*, **55**, 1–33.

11. Wands, J.R. (2004) Prevention of hepatocellular carcinoma. *The New England Journal of Medicine*, **351**, 1567–1570.

12. Wasley, A., Grytdal, S. & Gallagher, K. (2008) Surveillance for acute viral hepatitis – United States, 2006. *MMWR Surveillance Summaries*, **57**, 1–24.

13. Judd, A., Hickman, M., Hope, V.D., *et al.* (2007) Twenty years of selective hepatitis B vaccination: Is hepatitis B declining among injecting drug users in England and Wales? *Journal of Viral Hepatitis*, **14**, 584–591.

14. Alter, M.J., Margolis, H.S., Krawczynski, K., *et al.* (1992) The natural history of community-acquired hepatitis C in the United States. *The New England Journal of Medicine*, **327**, 1899–1905.

15. Liaw, Y.F. (1995) Role of hepatitis C virus in dual and triple hepatitis virus infection. *Hepatology*, **22**, 1101–1108.

16. Zignego, A.L., Fontana, R., Puliti, S., *et al.* (1997) Relevance of inapparent coinfection by hepatitis B virus in alpha interferon-treated patients with hepatitis C virus chronic hepatitis. *Journal of Medical Virology*, **51**, 313–318.

17. McMahon, J.M., Pouget, E.R. & Tortu, S. (2007) Individual and couple-level risk factors for hepatitis C infection among heterosexual drug users: A multilevel dyadic analysis. *Journal of Infectious Diseases*, **195**, 1572–1581.

18. Prati, D. (2006) Transmission of hepatitis C virus by blood transfusions and other medical procedures: A global review. *Journal of Hepatology*, **45**, 607–616.

19. Mazzaro, C., Tirelli, U. & Pozzato, G. (2005) Hepatitis C virus and non-Hodgkin's lymphoma 10 years later. *Digestive and Liver Disease*, **37**, 219–226.

20. Wiwanitkit, V. (2007) Hepatitis virus infection and Hodgkin's lymphoma: A review of the literature. *Hepatitis Monthly*, **7**, 229–231.

21. Greco-Stewart, V.S., Miron, P., Abrahem, A. & Pelchat, M. (2007) The human RNA polymerase II interacts with the terminal stem-loop regions of the hepatitis delta virus RNA genome. *Virology*, **357**, 68–78.

22. Oyunsuren, T., Kurbanov, F., Tanaka, Y., *et al.* (2006) High frequency of hepatocellular carcinoma in Mongolia; association with mono-, or co-infection with hepatitis C, B, and delta viruses. *Journal of Medical Virology*, **78**, 1688–1695.

23. IARC (1994) Hepatitis D virus. *IARC Monographs on the Evaluation of Carcinogenic Risks to Humans*, **59**, 223. International Agency for Research on Cancer, Lyon.

24. Yang, J.F., Dai, C.Y., Chuang, W.L., *et al.* (2006) Prevalence and clinical significance of HGV/GBV-C infection in patients with chronic hepatitis B or C. *Japanese Journal of Infectious Diseases*, **59**, 25–30.

25. Bosch, F.X. & Iftner, T. (2005) Papillomavirus. In: *The Aetiology of Cervical Cancer*, pp. 3–16. NHS Cancer Screening Programmes, Sheffield.

26. Centers for Disease Control and Prevention. (2007) *Human Papillomavirus: HPV Information for Clinicians*. Centers for Disease Control and Prevention, U.S.Department of Health and Human Services, Atlanta, GA.

27. Hampl, M. (2007) Prevention of human papilloma virus-induced preneoplasia and cancer by prophylactic HPV vaccines. *Minerva Medica*, **98**, 121–130.

28. Walboomers, J.M., Jacobs, M.V., Manos, M.M., Bosch, F.X., Kummer, J.A. & Shah, K.V. (1999) Human papillomavirus is a necessary cause of invasive cervical cancer worldwide. *Journal of Pathology*, **189**, 12–19.

29. Steben, M. & Duarte-Franco, E. (2007) Human papillomavirus infection: Epidemiology and pathophysiology. *Gynecologic Oncology*, **107**, S2–S5.

30. Dehn, D., Torkko, K.C. & Shroyer, K.R. (2007) Human papillomavirus testing and molecular markers of cervical dysplasia and carcinoma. *Cancer*, **111**, 1–14.

31. American College of Obstetricians and Gynecologists. (2003) ACOG Practice Bulletin: Clinical management guidelines for obstetrician-gynecologists. Number 45, August 2003. Cervical cytology screening (replaces committee opinion 152, March 1995). *Obstetrics & Gynecology*, **102**, 417–427.

32. LeBoit, P.E., Burg, G., Weedon, D. & Sarasain, A. (2006) Keratinocytic tumours. In: *World Health Organization Classification of Tumours. Pathology and Genetics of Skin Tumours* (eds P.E. LeBoit, G. Burg, D. Weedon & A. Sarasain), pp. 9–48. IARC Press, Lyon.

33. Hoory, T., Monie, A., Gravitt, P. & Wu, T.-C. (2008) Molecular epidemiology of human papillomavirus. *Journal of the Formosan Medical Association*, **107**, 198–217.

34. Bosch, F.X., Rohan, T., Schneider, A., *et al.* (2001) Papillomavirus research update: Highlights of the Barcelona HPV 2000 international papillomavirus conference. *Journal of Clinical Pathology*, **54**, 163–175.

35. Boukamp, P. (2005) Non-melanoma skin cancer: What drives tumor development and progression? *Carcinogenesis*, **26**, 1657–1667.

36. Psyrri, A. & DiMaio, D. (2008) Human papillomavirus in cervical and head-and-neck cancer. *Nature Clinical Practice Oncology*, **5**, 24–31.

37. Applebaum, K.M., Furniss, C.S., Zeka, A., *et al.* (2007) Lack of association of alcohol and tobacco with HPV16-associated head and neck cancer. *Journal of the National Cancer Institute*, **99**, 1801–1810.

38. D'Souza, G., Kreimer, A.R., Viscidi, R., *et al.* (2007) Case-control study of human papillomavirus and oropharyngeal cancer. *The New England Journal of Medicine*, **356**, 1944–1956.

39. Lever, A.M. & Berkhout, B. (2008) 2008 Nobel prize in medicine for discoverers of HIV. *Retrovirology*, **5**, 91.

40. Uchiyama, T., Yodoi, J., Sagawa, K., Takatsuki, K. & Uchino, H. (1977) Adult T-cell leukemia: Clinical and hematologic features of 16 cases. *Blood*, **50**, 481–492.

41. Poiesz, B.J., Ruscetti, F.W., Gazdar, A.F., Bunn, P.A., Minna, J.D. & Gallo, R.C. (1980) Detection and isolation of type C retrovirus particles from fresh and cultured lymphocytes of a patient with cutaneous T-cell lymphoma. *Proceedings of the National Academy of Sciences USA*, **77**, 7415–7419.

42. Kalyanaraman, V.S., Sarngadharan, M.G., Nakao, Y., Ito, Y., Aoki, T. & Gallo, R.C. (1982) Natural antibodies to the structural core protein (p24) of the human T-cell leukemia (lymphoma) retrovirus found in sera of leukemia patients in Japan. *Proceedings of the National Academy of Sciences USA*, **79**, 1653–1657.

43. Tokudome, S., Tokunaga, O., Shimamoto, Y., *et al.* (1989) Incidence of adult T-cell leukemia/lymphoma among human T-lymphotropic virus type I carriers in Saga, Japan. *Cancer Research*, **49**, 226–228.

44. IARC. (1996) Human immunodeficiency viruses and human T-cell lymphotropic viruses. *IARC Monographs on the Evaluation of Carcinogenic Risks to Humans*, **67**, 31–38. International Agency for Research on Cancer, Lyon.

45. Verdonck, K., Gonzalez, E., Van Dooren, S., Vandamme, A.M., Vanham, G. & Gotuzzo, E. (2007) Human T-lymphotropic virus 1: Recent knowledge of an ancient infection. *The Lancet Infectious Diseases*, **7**, 266–281.

46. Sarid, R., Klepfish, A. & Schattner, A. (2002) Virology, pathogenetic mechanisms, and associated diseases of Kaposi sarcoma-associated herpesvirus (human herpesvirus 8). *Mayo Clinic Proceedings*, **77**, 941–949.

47. Schulz, T.F. (1999) Epidemiology of Kaposi's sarcoma-associated herpesvirus/human herpesvirus 8. *Advances in Cancer Research*, **76**, 121–160.

48. Kaposi, M. (1982) Idiopathic multiple pigmented sarcoma of the skin (Trans. from *Archives of Dermatology and Syphilology*, **4**, 265–272, 1872). *Archives of Dermatology and Syphilology*, **32**, 342–347.

49. Kaposi, M. (1872) Idiopathisches multiples Pigmentsarkom der Haut. *Archiv für Dermatologie und Syphilis*, **4**, 265–272.

50. Calonje, E. (2002) Vascular tumours. In: *Pathology and Genetics of Tumours of Soft Tissue and Bone* (eds C.D.M. Fletcher, K.K. Unni & F. Mertens), pp. 155–178. IARC Press, Lyon.

51. Guttman-Yassky, E., Cohen, A., Kra-Oz, Z., *et al.* (2004) Familial clustering of classic Kaposi sarcoma. *Journal of Infectious Diseases*, **189**, 2023–2026.

52. Szajerka, T. & Jablecki, J. (2007) Kaposi's sarcoma revisited. *AIDS Reviews*, **9**, 3–10.

53. Ziegler, J.L. (1993) Endemic Kaposi's sarcoma in Africa and local volcanic soils. *Lancet*, **342**, 1348–1351.

54. Davey, G., Tekola, F. & Newport, M.J. (2007) Podoconiosis: Non-infectious geochemical elephantiasis. *Transactions of the Royal Society of Tropical Medicine and Hygiene*, **101**, 1175–1180.

55. Price, E.W. & Henderson, W.J. (1978) The elemental content of lymphatic tissues in barefooted people in Ethiopia, with reference to endemic elephantiasis of the lower legs. *Transactions of the Royal Society of Tropical Medicine and Hygiene*, **72**, 132–136.

56. Ziegler, J.L., Simonart, T. & Snoeck, R. (2001) Kaposi's sarcoma, oncogenic viruses, and iron. *Journal of Clinical Virology*, **20**, 127–130.

57. Abrahams, P.W. (2002) Soils: Their implications to human health. *Science of the Total Environment*, **291**, 1–32.

58. Montagnino, G., Bencini, P.L., Tarantino, A., *et al.* (1994) Clinical features and course of Kaposi's sarcoma in kidney transplant patients: Report of 13 cases. *American Journal of Nephrology*, **14**, 121–126.

59. Harwood, A.R., Osaba, D., Hofstader, S.L., *et al.* (1979) Kaposi's sarcoma in recipients of renal transplants. *American Journal of Medicine*, **67**, 759–765.

60. Mendez, J.C. & Paya, C.V. (2000) Kaposi's sarcoma and transplantation. *Herpes*, **7**, 18–23.

61. Engels, E.A., Biggar, R.J., Hall, H.I., *et al.* (2008) Cancer risk in people infected with human immunodeficiency virus in the United States. *International Journal of Cancer*, **123**, 187–194.

62. Travis, W.D., Brambilla, E., Muller-Hermelink, H.K. & Harris, C.C. (2004) Tumours of the pleura. In: *World Health Organization Classification of Tumours. Pathology and Genetics of Tumours of the Lung, Pleura, Thymus and Heart* (eds W.D. Travis, E. Brambilia, H.K. Muller-Hermelink & C.C. Harris), pp. 125–144. IARC Press, Lyon.

63. Kroczynska, B., Cutrone, R., Bocchetta, M., *et al.* (2006) Crocidolite asbestos and SV40 are cocarcinogens in human mesothelial cells and in causing mesothelioma in hamsters. *Proceedings of the National Academy of Sciences USA*, **103**, 14128–14133.

64. Hahn, W.C. & Weinberg, R.A. (2002) Rules for making human tumor cells. *The New England Journal of Medicine*, **347**, 1593–1603.

65. Leithner, K., Leithner, A., Clar, H., *et al.* (2006) Mesothelioma mortality in Europe: Impact of asbestos consumption and simian virus 40. *Orphanet Journal of Rare Diseases*, **1**, 44.

66. Peto, J., Hodgson, J.T., Matthews, F.E. & Jones, J.R. (1995) Continuing increase in mesothelioma mortality in Britain. *Lancet*, **345**, 535–539.

67. Becker, J.C., Schrama, D. & Houben, R. (2009) Merkel cell carcinoma. *Cellular and Molecular Life Sciences*, **66**, 1–8.

68. Heymann, W.R. (2008) Merkel cell carcinoma: Insights into pathogenesis. *Journal of the American Academy of Dermatology*, **59**, 503–504.

69. Feng, H., Shuda, M., Chang, Y. & Moore, P.S. (2008) Clonal integration of a polyomavirus in human Merkel cell carcinoma. *Science*, **319**, 1096–1100.

70. Schmidt, C. (2008) Yuan Chang and Patrick Moore: Teaming up to hunt down cancer-causing viruses. *Journal of the National Cancer Institute*, **100**, 524–525, 529.

71. zur Hausen, H. (2008) Novel human polyomaviruses – Re-emergence of a well known virus family as possible human carcinogens. *International Journal of Cancer*, **123**, 247–250.

72. Linz, B., Balloux, F., Moodley, Y., *et al.* (2007) An African origin for the intimate association between humans and *Helicobacter pylori*. *Nature*, **445**, 915–918.

73. Eppinger, M., Baar, C., Linz, B., *et al.* (2006) Who ate whom? Adaptive Helicobacter genomic changes that accompanied a host jump from early humans to large felines. *PLoS Genetics*, **2**, e120.

74. Marshall, B.J. (1993) *Helicobacter pylori*: A primer for 1994. *Gastroenterologist*, **1**, 241–247.

75. Kivi, M. & Tindberg, Y. (2006) *Helicobacter pylori* occurrence and transmission: A family affair? *Scandinavian Journal of Infectious Diseases*, **38**, 407–417.

76. Czinn, S.J. (2005) *Helicobacter pylori* infection: Detection, investigation, and management. *Journal of Pediatrics*, **146**, S21–S26.

77. Boffetta, P. (1997) Infection with *Helicobacter pylori* and parasites, social class and cancer. In: *Social Inequalities and Cancer* (eds M. Kogavinas, N. Pearce, M. Susser & P. Boffetta), pp. 325–329. International Agency for Research on Cancer, Lyon.

78. Logan, R.P. & Walker, M.M. (2001) ABC of the upper gastrointestinal tract: Epidemiology and diagnosis of *Helicobacter pylori* infection. *British Medical Journal*, **323**, 920–922.

79. Sonnenberg, A. (2006) Causes underlying the birth-cohort phenomenon of peptic ulcer: Analysis of mortality data 1911–2000, England and Wales. *International Journal of Epidemiology*, **35**, 1090–1097.

80. Jacobson, K. (2005) The changing prevalence of *Helicobacter pylori* infection in Canadian children: Should screening be performed in high-risk children? *Canadian Journal of Gastroenterology*, **19**, 412–414.

81. Blaser, M.J. (2006) Who are we? Indigenous microbes and the ecology of human diseases. *EMBO Reports*, **7**, 956–960.

82. McMahon, B.J., Bruce, M.G., Hennessy, T.W., *et al.* (2006) Reinfection after successful eradication of *Helicobacter pylori*: A 2-year prospective study in Alaska Natives. *Alimentary Pharmacology and Therapeutics*, **23**, 1215–1223.

83. Wu, M.S., Chen, C.J. & Lin, J.T. (2005) Host-environment interactions: Their impact on progression from gastric inflammation to carcinogenesis and on development of new approaches to prevent and treat gastric cancer. *Cancer Epidemiology, Biomarkers & Prevention*, **14**, 1878–1882.

84. Kamangar, F., Dawsey, S.M., Blaser, M.J., *et al.* (2006) Opposing risks of gastric cardia and non-cardia gastric adenocarcinomas associated with *Helicobacter pylori* seropositivity. *Journal of the National Cancer Institute*, **98**, 1445–1452.

85. Lagergren, J. (2006) Etiology and risk factors for oesophageal adenocarcinoma: Possibilities for chemoprophylaxis? *Best Practice & Research Clinical Gastroenterology*, **20**, 803–812.

86. Du, M.Q. & Wotherspoon, A.C. (2002) Gastric MALT lymphoma: From aetiology to treatment. *Lancet Oncology*, **3**, 97–104.

87. Leung, W.K. & Sung, J.J. (2006) Chemoprevention of gastric cancer. *European Journal of Gastroenterology & Hepatology*, **18**, 867–871.

88. Yang, L. (2006) Incidence and mortality of gastric cancer in China. *World Journal of Gastroenterology*, **12**, 17–20.

89. Allan, F., Rollinson, D., Smith, J.E. & Dunn, A.M. (2009) Host choice and penetration by *Schistosoma haematobium* miracidia. *Journal of Helminthology*, **83**, 33–38.

90. Gryseels, B., Polman, K., Clerinx, J. & Kestens, L. (2006) Human schistosomiasis. *Lancet*, **368**, 1106–1118.

91. Dunne, D.W. & Cooke, A. (2005) A worm's eye view of the immune system: Consequences for evolution of human autoimmune disease. *Nature Reviews Immunology*, **5**, 420–426.

92. IARC. (1994) Schistosomes, liver flukes and *Helicobacter pylori*. IARC working group on the evaluation of carcinogenic risks to humans. Lyon, 7–14 June 1994. *IARC Monographs on the Evaluation of Carcinogenic Risks to Humans*, **61**, 1–241. International Agency for Research on Cancer, Lyon.

93. Pearce, E.J. & MacDonald, A.S. (2002) The immunobiology of schistosomiasis. *Nature Reviews Immunology*, **2**, 499–511.

94. Whitfield, D., Curtis, C.F., White, G.B., Targett, G.A.T., Warhurst, D.C. & Bradley, D.J. (1984) Two cases of falciparum malaria acquired in Britain. *British Medical Journal*, **289**, 1607–1609.

95. Khurana, S., Dubey, M.L. & Malla, N. (2005) Association of parasitic infections and cancers. *Indian Journal of Medical Microbiology*, **23**, 74–79.

96. RBM/WHO/UNICEF. (2005) *World Malaria Report*. RBM/WHO/UNICEF, Geneva.

97. Hatz, C.F. (2006) Schistosomiasis: An underestimated problem in industrialized countries? *Journal of Travel Medicine*, **12**, 1.

98. Ruffer, M.A. (1910) Note on the presence of "Bilharzia haematobia" in Egyptian mummies of the twentieth dynasty (1250–1000 B.C.). *British Medical Journal*, **1**, 16.

99. Pisani, P., Parkin, D.M., Munoz, N. & Ferlay, J. (1997) Cancer and infection: Estimates of the attributable fraction in 1990. *Cancer Epidemiology, Biomarkers & Prevention*, **6**, 387–400.

100. Day, J.H., Grant, A.D., Doherty, J.F., Chiodini, P.L. & Wright, S.G. (1996) Schistosomiasis in travellers returning from sub-Saharan Africa. *British Medical Journal*, **313**, 268–269.

101. Whitty, C.J., Mabey, D.C., Armstrong, M., *et al.* (2000) Presentation and outcome of 1107 cases of schistosomiasis from Africa diagnosed in a non-endemic country. *Transactions of the Royal Society of Tropical Medicine and Hygiene*, **94**, 531–534.

102. Health Protection Agency. (2007) *Foreign Travel-associated Illness in England, Wales and Northern Ireland: 2007 Report*. Health Protection Agency, London.

103. Chai, J.Y., Murrell, K.D. & Lymbery, A.J. (2005) Fish-borne parasitic zoonoses: Status and issues. *International Journal for Parasitology*, **35**, 1233–1254.

104. Parkin, D.M., Ohshima, H., Srivatanakul, P. & Vatanasapt, V. (1993) Cholangiocarcinoma: Epidemiology, mechanisms of carcinogenesis and prevention. *Cancer Epidemiology, Biomarkers & Prevention*, **2**, 537–544.

105. Srivatanakul, P., Ohshima, H., Khlat, M., *et al.* (1991) *Opisthorchis viverrini* infestation and endogenous nitrosamines as risk factors for cholangiocarcinoma in Thailand. *International Journal of Cancer*, **48**, 821–825.

106. Bartsch, H., Ohshima, H., Pignatelli, B. & Calmels, S. (1992) Endogenously formed N-nitroso compounds and nitrosating agents in human cancer etiology. *Pharmacogenetics*, **2**, 272–277.

107. Mitacek, E.J., Brunnemann, K.D., Hoffmann, D., *et al.* (1999) Volatile nitrosamines and tobacco-specific nitrosamines in the smoke of Thai cigarettes: A risk factor for lung cancer and a suspected risk factor for liver cancer in Thailand. *Carcinogenesis*, **20**, 133–137.

108. Keiser, J. & Utzinger, J. (2005) Emerging foodborne trematodiasis. *Emerging Infectious Diseases*, **11**, 1507–1514.

109. Health Protection Agency. (2006) *Migrant Health: Infectious Diseases in Non-UK Born Populations in England, Wales and Northern Ireland. A Baseline Report – 2006.* Health Protection Agency Centre for Infections, London.

110. Yossepowitch, O., Gotesman, T., Assous, M., Marva, E., Zimlichman, R. & Dan, M. (2004) Opisthorchiasis from imported raw fish. *Emerging Infectious Diseases*, **10**, 2122–2126.

111. Stauffer, W.M., Sellman, J.S. & Walker, P.F. (2004) Biliary liver flukes (Opisthorchiasis and Clonorchiasis) in immigrants in the United States: Often subtle and diagnosed years after arrival. *Journal of Travel Medicine*, **11**, 157–159.

112. Patel, T. (2002) Worldwide trends in mortality from biliary tract malignancies. *BMC Cancer*, **2**, 77–82.

113. Koch, R. (1882) Die Aetiologie der tuberkulose. *Berliner Klinischen Wochenschrift*, **15**, 221–230.

114. McLaughlin-Drubin, M.E. & Munger, K. (2008) Viruses associated with human cancer. *Biochimica et Biophysica Acta*, **1782**, 127–150.

115. Evans, A.S. & Mueller, N.E. (1990) Viruses and cancer. Causal associations. *Annals of Epidemiology*, **1**, 71–92.

116. Carbone, M., Klein, G., Gruber, J. & Wong, M. (2004) Modern criteria to establish human cancer etiology. *Cancer Research*, **64**, 5518–5524.

117. Pagano, J.S., Blaser, M., Buendia, M.A., *et al.* (2004) Infectious agents and cancer: Criteria for a causal relation. *Seminars in Cancer Biology*, **14**, 453–471.

118. Woodhouse, M.E., Howey, R., Gaunt, E., Reilly, I., Chase-Toppping, M. & Savill, N. (2008) Temporal trends in the discovery of human viruses. *Proceedings of the Royal Society B: Biological Sciences*, **275**, 2111–2115.

3 Molecular biology of cancer

The assumption is made in the essay that the reader is familiar with basic concepts of molecular biology such as the role of DNA, the nature of the gene, etc. For an introduction to such concepts a variety of web sites and books[1,2] are available, and journal review articles are often readily accessible[3,4].

Key events in malignant transformation

The key features of a malignant clone are:

- Immortality – the cells do not mature and do not die
- Independence – the clone does not rely on signals from other cells to survive or to divide
- Mobility – the defining feature for malignant versus benign tumours is the ability of the former to violate boundaries between anatomical compartments and to seed remote colonies (metastases)
- Subversion – malignant tumours inhibit components of the immune system, and may influence non-malignant cells to create a favourable milieu for the cancer cell, for example, cytokines produced by myeloma regulate behaviour of osteoblasts and osteoclasts
- Instability – although it is not a defining feature, it is a characteristic of virtually all malignancies that they spin off ever more genetically aberrant sub-clones
- Angiogenesis induction – malignant tumours, and possibly some benign tumours such as haemangiomas, have the capacity to induce the growth of new blood vessels to nourish the developing tumour

It is an extraordinary fact that, as long ago as 1914, a scientist named Theodore Boveri recognized the key features of malignant cells[5]:

Infectious Causes of Cancer, first edition. By Ken Campbell. Published 2011 by John Wiley & Sons Ltd.
© 2011 John Wiley & Sons Ltd.

■ Cell-cycle checkpoints (Hemmungseinrichtung: inhibitory mechanism) that would allow cell division only when a specific external stimulus is experienced by the cell.

■ Tumour-suppressor genes (Teilungshemmende Chromosomen), the effects of which can be overcome by external signals, and which are physically lost in progressively growing tumours.

■ Oncogenes (Teilungsfoerdernde Chromosomen) that become amplified (im permanenten bergewicht) during tumour development.

■ Tumour progression from benign to malignant, involving sequential changes of increased growth-stimulatory chromosomes and loss of growth-inhibitory chromosomes.

■ The clonal origin of tumours.

■ Genetic mosaicism.

■ Cancer predisposition through inheritance of chromosomes (genes) that are less able to suppress malignancy.

■ Cancer predisposition through inheritance of genes that cause aberrant mitoses.

■ Inheritance of the same 'weak chromosome' from both parents leads to homozygosity for the defective chromosome and, consequently, to high-penetrance cancer syndromes – for example, xeroderma pigmentosum.

■ The role of wounding and inflammation in tumour promotion.

■ Loss of cell adhesion in metastasis.

■ Sensitivity of malignant cells to radiation therapy.

In a remarkable series of experiments, it was shown that a minimum of four genes must have been malfunctioning for a cell to undergo malignant transformation[6]. The only one of these elements Boveri had not foreseen was the importance of telomerase; he had no way of knowing of the existence of structures called telomeres on the ends of chromosomes, which prevent unravelling of the DNA molecule. The next section will, very briefly, recap the features of normal controls on cell growth, maturation, division and death.

The normal background to malignant transformation

Apoptosis

In 1972, Kerr, Wylie and Currie first described and named the process of apoptosis – often referred to as programmed cell death[7,8]. Kerr and his colleagues had recognized that, in multicellular organisms there were at least two distinct forms of cell death. In necrosis a whole group of neighbouring cells die, in so doing they spill out their contents which excites an inflammatory response. In apoptosis, in contrast, an individual cell neatly packages its internal contents, breaks down its DNA and then displays markers on its surface inviting phagocytic cells of the immune system to come and clear away the debris. There is no inflammatory response to apoptosis and, far from being pathological it is a vital physiological process. Apoptosis is vital in the moulding of primitive embryonic limb buds into arms and legs; it regulates the conversion of a mass of callus at the site of a fracture into a normally shaped and functioning bone. Most vitally in our context, apoptosis is the mechanism by which the body eliminates cells which have acquired defects in their genome – this is a vital part of the defences against cancer. There are several apoptosis-based anti-cancer agents currently under development; although most cancer therapies depend to some extent on induction of apoptotic pathways these are therapies designed specifically to trigger apoptotic pathways.

It has long been accepted that, with the possible exception of some paediatric cancers, it is necessary for multiple independent genetic lesions to occur in regions of the genome regulating cell growth, division and death[9]. In the human genome there are approximately 3 billion base pairs which must be accurately replicated each time a cell divides. A sophisticated proofreading and error correction pathway ensure the accuracy of this process. The process is so accurate that the 3 billion base pair genome will only change by about 10–20 bases a year[10]. A back-up system to ensure the integrity of the genome assesses errors and the success of the dividing cell in correcting these; if the cell fails this assessment the apoptosis pathways are triggered and the cell self-destructs. It is only if both the DNA repair and the apoptosis pathways are defective or suppressed that a cell can become malignant.

Entry into cell cycle

Three major types of tissues can be recognized in adults – labile, stable and permanent[11].

- Labile tissues are those in which there is a high rate of cell loss and, consequently, of cell production – tissues such as blood and epithelial linings. The functional mature cells have a set, usually brief, life-span and therefore their stem cell populations divide throughout life.
- Stable tissues, such as liver, have mature end-stage cells with a long life span and a low rate of attrition in the absence of disease or injury. These tissues contain stem cell populations which are normally quiescent or minimally active, but which have the capacity to divide rapidly if replenishment is necessary.
- Permanent tissues, such as neurons or cardiac muscle, have been thought to have little or no stem cell compartment. Cells can recover from sub-lethal damage but the potential for cell replacement in adult life has been presumed to be absent or very limited. (Although the inclusion of a permanent category is still useful, there is increasing awareness that the distinction is not absolute and these tissues do have stem cell populations and some capacity for repair and regeneration in adult life[12].)

Even in labile tissues most stem cells are quiescent at any given time; end-stage mature functional cells have, in the process of maturation, lost their capacity for division. A colossal number of new cells is required daily to replace those lost through senility, or by attrition at interfaces with the outside world; the skin, the lining of the gut and respiratory tract, and the lining of the urogenital tract. These cells are replaced by exponential expansion from a limited pool of pluripotent stem cells – it has been proposed that there may be a single pool from which all peripheral stem cell populations are replenished[13]. It is this very potential for exponential expansion that allows the progeny of one rogue cell to produce a malignant tumour that ultimately threatens the host organism's survival.

Under normal circumstances there is a series of restraints on cell growth and replication. Cells behave cooperatively; even the continued survival of a cell depends on the receipt of regulatory signals from its neighbours. All cells in humans are primed to undergo apoptosis, a genetically programmed process of orderly self-destruction. Apoptosis is of great importance in organ modelling during foetal development, in organ remodelling and tissue repair during adult life, in eliminating self-reacting clones in the immune system and in many other aspects of healthy growth and development. Inhibition of the apoptotic process depends on a continuous stream of signals from outside the cell. One of the earliest events in malignant transformation is suppression of the apoptotic pathways.

It is axiomatic that in multi-celled organisms no normal cell may arbitrarily decide to divide – the explicit consent of at least one neighbour is required. For a normal cell to undergo division it must receive a triggering, or at least permissive, signal from another cell. The binding of the growth factor to a surface growth factor receptor triggers a sequence of events, via intracellular messenger proteins, with activation of cell-cycle genes initiating the process of DNA copying and cell division. Another crucial event in malignant transformation is the achievement of independence from the requirement for an external growth factor signal.

The cell cycle

When cells divide they do so in an ordered sequence under the control of genes, which are highly conserved across species as diverse as yeasts and humans. All of the genes regulating cell, division, maturation, growth and death are highly conserved. This indicates that they arose early in the evolutionary process and that their normal functioning is fundamental to the survival of any multi-celled organism. They have undergone so little change over evolution that one can transfer yeast genes into a human cell and they will function normally.

The cell cycle is a sequence of stages during which DNA is copied, the fidelity of that copying is checked, the cell repairs any errors (or undergoes apoptosis if they are irreparable), and finally the new DNA must be packaged into chromosomes and distributed within the cell such that each daughter cell will receive an appropriate complement. All this takes a matter of some hours in the normal cell, perhaps paradoxically, in cancer cells the division time is frequently prolonged as shown in the Table 3.1[14].

Table 3.1   Time taken to complete cell cycle

Cell type	Hours
Normal Cells	
Bone marrow precursor cells	18
Lining cells of large intestine	39
Lining cells of rectum	48
Fertilized ovum	36–60
Cancer cells	
Stomach	72
Chronic myeloid leukaemia	120
Lung (bronchial carcinoma)	196–260

There are four stages in cell division:

■ G1 phase – the cell grows in size
■ S phase – the chromosomes are replicated
■ G2 phase – further growth and preparation for division
■ M phase – in which the nucleus and then the cell divide to produce two daughter cells

The large majority of cells, which are not dividing or preparing to divide, are in G0 or rest phase. Entry into and progress through the cell cycle are controlled by a constellation of regulatory compounds called cyclins – these in turn transmit their messages through subordinate proteins called cyclin-dependent kinases (CDKs).

A detailed discussion of the machinery of cell division is beyond the scope of this chapter – a good account can be found in any standard cell biology textbook or on the web by searching for 'cell cycle'.

The Hayflick limit

When cells are cultured in vitro, there is a limit to the number of cell divisions which they can undergo. This is referred to as the Hayflick limit, after the scientist who first described the phenomenon[15]. This is thought to relate to telomere biology – telomeres are repeated DNA sequences found at the end of chromosomes[16], they have been likened to the metal tags of the end of shoelaces. They protect chromosome ends from fusion, combination or being seen as damaged DNA. Each time a cell divides the telomere shortens by about 100 bases, this is because the DNA polymerase enzymes cannot replicate to the very end of a DNA strand. When telomeres shorten beyond a certain point the cell undergoes apoptosis. The only exceptions under normal circumstances are stem cells and germ cells. These cell populations possess an enzyme called telomerase which can extend the telomeric region – acquisition of telomerase activity by cancer cells contributes to their immortalization. It has been shown that tumour viruses have evolved several different ways to subvert this check on cell division[17].

Malignant transformation

The process of malignant transformation requires a single cell to acquire a complex of genetic changes, which allow that cell to subvert normal controls regulating cell growth, division and death. In addition, the cell must escape from localization controls, which would normally prevent the cell from breaching basement membrane integrity and from establishing metastases. Cancer genes can essentially be grouped into three major types; these are often described by analogy to a runaway vehicle:

■ Oncogenes – which drive pathological cell division – the accelerator
■ Tumour suppressor genes – which normally inhibit growth and division – the brakes
■ DNA repair genes – responsible for maintaining genomic integrity – the incompetent mechanic

Telomerase is necessary to permit the cell to attain immortality; this gene is in a category of its own, it is normally only expressed in stem cells and in germ cells (ova and sperm).

Types of chromosome abnormality

There is a relatively limited spectrum of ways in which the genome may become deranged. The exact defects may affect almost any part of any chromosomes but they all fall into a limited number of categories. An excellent account of the genetics of haematological malignancies can be found in *Essential Haematology*[18]; despite its haematological bias, the general principles apply to all cancers.

Quantitative anomalies

Aneuploidy
Normal human cells contain a complement of 22 pairs of autosomal chromosomes and one pair of sex chromosomes. The full complement of 46 chromosomes is found in all cells except gametes (sperm and ova), which contain half the full number. The full set of 46 chromosomes is said to be the diploid complement, while a half set is the haploid number. A cell that contains an incorrect number of chromosomes is said to be aneuploid. Aneuploidy is a very common feature of cancer cells.

Aneuploidy may involve acquisition of additional copies of a gene – one of the best-known examples of this is Down syndrome or trisomy 21 in which there are three instead of two copies of chromosome 21. Trisomy 12 is often seen in chronic lymphocytic leukaemia – it tends to be associated with a poorer prognosis than for patients who do not have this specific defect. Alternatively, cancer cells may be missing a copy of a particular chromosome – chromosome 5 and chromosome 7 are each often only present as a single copy in patients with myelodysplastic syndrome. Again the abnormality tends to have prognostic significance. There is a form of MDS in which absence of the whole of chromosome 5 is associated with distinctive clinical features – this is called 5q-syndrome and carries a good prognosis.

Amplification/deletion
Aneuploidy is an extreme example of a more general phenomenon – gain or loss of genetic material. In its most subtle form this may be duplication of a single gene or loss of a single tumour suppressor gene. For the purpose of describing sections of a chromosome the abbreviation q refers to the long arm and the abbreviation p refers to the short arm. Thus, 5q- would refer to deletion of the entire long arm of chromosome 5. A more detailed description may be given when only part of a chromosome arm is deleted, for example del(7)(q31q32).

Viral genetic insertion
A special case of acquisition of genetic material occurs when a virus inserts genetic material into the genome of a cell – this is called transfection. Transfection of blood stem cells has been used as a therapy for a condition called SCID in which there is near total loss of the immune defences. Unfortunately, of the small numbers of patients in whom this has so far been attempted, two have developed a leukaemia-like syndrome. This has led to some calls for a complete moratorium on use of the technique until it is better understood how viruses insert their material.

Loss of heterozygosity/loss of imprinting
It has been discovered that in many genes only one of the two copies present is functional. In some cases this is the paternal copy, in others the maternal copy. The process by which one copy is switched off is called imprinting. It is currently estimated that as few as 100 of the 30 000 or so genes in humans shows imprinting – the impact is however great because many of the affected genes are either tumour suppressor genes or oncogenes.

Where genes show imprinting, an additional mechanism is open for carcinogenic transformation of the genome. If we are considering a tumour suppressor gene (a brake on cell division), if the only functional copy is switched off, this alone will not suffice to cause cancer but it may contribute to the process. In an oncogene (a gene-driving cell division forward), switching on of both copies may drive a cell to divide in the absence of appropriate external signals. A fact sheet on imprinting can be found at http://www.genetics.com.au/pdf/factsheets/fs15.pdf. In some cases, loss of imprinting occurs when maternal and paternal copies of a gene are present but imprinting is defective. In other instances, a cell has received two copies of either the paternal or the maternal gene, instead of one of each – this is termed loss of heterozygosity.

Qualitative anomalies

An alternative form of anomaly exists, in which the number of chromosomes is normal and there is no significant gain or loss of genetic material, but in which portions of genetic material have been transferred from their proper site to a different location. Where this involves exchange of material between sites, usually on different chromosomes, it is called a translocation.

Translocations

Balanced translocations involve transfer of genetic material between two or more chromosomes – these may be very complex involving large-scale transfer of genes between chromosomes but without gains or losses. In an unbalanced translocation, there is both a qualitative and a quantitative defect or defects. There is transfer of genetic material but there is also a net gain or loss of genetic material.

Translocations may lead to production of a novel fusion gene not seen in nature, or they may lead to a functional gene coming under the influence of an inappropriate control gene. An example of the former is the first chromosome abnormality recognized to be associated with a specific cancer – the Philadelphia chromosome and chronic myeloid leukaemia. This results from translocation of a portion of chromosome 9 onto chromosome 22. This is a balanced translocation with part of chromosome 22 found on chromosome 9, but the leukaemogenic fusion gene is found on the abnormal chromosome 22. The gene ABL (Abelson oncogene) on chromosome 9 is fused with the gene BCR (Breakpoint Cluster Region) on chromosome 22. This produces a tyrosine kinase which is constantly switched on and which drives cell division and other aspects of malignant transformation. The latter example may involve switching off of a tumour suppressor gene, allowing the cancer cell free rein; or alternatively, it may involve continuous expression of a growth-promoting gene (an oncogene).

Inversion

This is similar in consequences to a translocation but involves a segment of a chromosome being re-inserted into the same chromosome in an inverted configuration. This can result in exactly the same forms of pathological recombination as for translocation –the difference is that the rearrangement occurs within the same chromosome.

Types of cancer gene

As mentioned above, there are basically three classes of cancer gene and one – telomerase – which stands in a class of its own.

Oncogenes

Oncogenes are genes that positively regulate cell growth and division – they cause a cell to enter cycle when it would not or they drive forwards the cell cycle. Oncogenes were first recognized as viral oncogenes – packages of genetic material carried by viruses, which, on insertion into a cell could initiate malignant disease. It was assumed that these must be foreign to the organism since such cancer-causing genes must be so dangerous. From the discovery by Peyton Rous of cancer causing viruses in the early twentieth century[19,20] it was to take 60 years before scientists were able to demonstrate which portions of the viral genome were oncogenes. To the surprise of those researchers the DNA sequences matched sequences found in normal mammalian cells. The sequences in viral genomes are now termed v-onc for viral oncogenes, while those in normal cells are called proto-oncogenes or cellular oncogenes – c-onc.

The normal genes matching the viral oncogenes were involved in control of cell division; they were also highly conserved across species suggesting that they may have been transferred into a virus that infected a cell in some distant ancestor of modern eukaryotes. An excellent discussion of viral oncogenes can be found in the textbook *Introduction to the Cellular and Molecular Biology of Cancer*[21].

Oncogenes, typically, act in a dominant fashion – in other words an abnormal, permanently active gene will override its normal counterpart and can contribute to malignant transformation. In contrast to these tumour suppressor genes, described below, normally require both copies to be defective or absent for a cancer to develop.

Oncogenes frequently code for proteins called tyrosine kinases – these are internal messengers, which act as intermediaries between the signal received by growth factor receptors at the cell surface and the sites within the nucleus where genes are switched in response to those growth signals. Usually, the normal function of an oncogene falls within one of four gene families:

■ Growth factors – genes for proteins circulating in the blood carrying messages between cells;
■ Cell surface receptors – genes coding for the molecules on cell surfaces which receive and pass on chemical messages from other cells;
■ Transcription factors – genes which regulate activity of genes by producing proteins which bind to those genes and switch them on or off; and
■ Signal transmission proteins – gene which regulate production of proteins that carry the signal from the cell surface receptors to the nucleus.

Growth factors are normally produced by one cell to regulate the behaviour of another cell(s) – if a cancer cell develops the ability to produce its own growth factors it becomes independent of external signals. Under normal circumstances there are three types of growth factor regulation:

■ Endocrine – in this form the growth factor is released into the circulation and regulates behaviour of distant cells;

■ Paracrine – in which the growth factor acts on a close neighbour of the secreting cell; and

■ Autocrine – when a cell releases a growth factor which can bind to receptors on the same cell – very few cells are able to do this under normal circumstances.

When a cell, which should be regulated by endocrine or paracrine growth factors, acquires the capacity for autocrine growth factor secretion it may become capable of autonomous division. In some cases cancer cells will secrete paracrine growth factors so that they stimulate each other's growth.

Tumour suppressor genes

Although Boveri foresaw their existence, Alfred Knudson's studies of retino-blastoma are generally credited with having established the concept of the anti-oncogene, now known as a tumour suppressor gene[22]. Where oncogenes drive forwards the cell cycle and cell division (the accelerator), tumour suppressor genes are negative regulators of cell division (the brakes). Appropriately for the analogy chosen, just like a car oncogenes typically can act independently, whereas tumour suppressor genes, like a car's multiple braking systems, operate cooperatively.

Tumour suppressor genes are necessary for the effective operation of DNA repair mechanisms. On proofreading of DNA, if anything above a minimal threshold of errors is met, pathways are initiated which put division on hold, while DNA repair is attempted. If repair is unsuccessful, the cell initiates apoptosis and sacrifices itself for the greater good. If tumour suppressor genes are absent or defective then arrest of the cell division process may fail to occur and the cell may generate a clone of faulty daughter cells, all of which share the same absence of functioning control mechanisms.

One of the most important tumour suppressor genes is called p53. This is the single most important gene in regulating the response to defective copying of DNA, in initiating the repair pathways and finally in ensuring apoptosis of any cell with an irreparably defective genome. For this reason p53 is sometimes called the 'guardian of the genome', and featured as 'Molecule of the year' in *Science* magazine in December 1993[23]. A detailed account of the biology of p53 can be found at *Online Mendelian Inheritance in Man, OMIM*™. Johns Hopkins University, Baltimore, Maryland. MIM Number: 191170: (2003): World Wide Web URL: http://www.ncbi.nlm.nih.gov/omim/191170; this is part of the US National Library of Medicine web site.

Other prominent examples of tumour suppressor genes are the genes BRCA1 and BRCA2 implicated in inherited breast cancer syndromes and retinoblastoma, already mentioned above.

DNA repair genes

Genomic instability is a virtually invariant feature of cancer cells – it has been cal-culated that a human lifetime would not be long enough for a cell to acquire a 'full set' of carcinogenic mutations at the background rate of mutation. If we assume that loss of stability of the genome is an early event in malignant transformation then the subsequent rate of accumulation of mutations will be much higher. As in other cases, the DNA repair genes are highly conserved across species implying that they emerged very early in eukaryote evolution and are of great importance to the cell. There are various different pathways to DNA repair, which pathway is activated depends on the exact nature of the defect in the DNA molecule. In some forms of DNA damage the two strands will no longer fit together – this is termed a DNA mismatch. The repair mechanism can identify the original (presumed cor-rect) strand because it carries methyl 'tags' which identify it – the daughter strand does not acquire these tags for some minutes after copying occurs. This is a long enough time frame for the repair machinery to compare the two strands and attempt to correct any errors detected.

A number of inherited conditions have been identified in which one, or several, of the DNA repair systems is defective. Affected individuals show a rate of cancer many times higher than background population rates. In particular they must take exquisite care to avoid exposure to the ultraviolet, DNA-damaging, components of the sun's radiation. Children with these conditions can only venture outdoors when clothed from head to foot in protective clothing. NASA has devised a lightweight suit which has, for the first time, given these children the freedom to play with their friends, although they must still be vigilant against any damage to the suit.

Angiogenesis

As tumours grow, their interiors become relatively ischaemic and, frequently, necrotic. They overcome the requirement for an oxygen and nutrient supply by releasing cytokines that trigger the development of new blood vessels. This has long been regarded as a potential target for anti-cancer therapy.

It is usually said that Judah Folkman, in Boston, was the first to suggest that growth of solid tumours beyond a few millimetres was dependent upon neovas-cularization, which in turn was induced by secretion of angiogenic factors. This had actually been proposed decades earlier in 1939 by Ide and colleagues who observed that transplanting a tumour into a rabbit's ear induced development of a complex vascular network and proposed that the tumour might produce a *'vessel growth-stimulating substance'*[24]. He further hypothesized that induction of angio-genesis, by offering access to the systemic vasculature, was a necessary precursor to metastatic spread. It was clear that this offered scope for development of thera-peutic agents. Almost 25 years later, in 1994, Judah Folkman and his team reported the development of an anti-angiogenic compound called Endostatin, which was effective at inhibiting new vessel development both in vitro and in murine models.

The initial response was hyperbole, particularly in the non-scientific press, which declared that the cure for all cancer was at hand. Folkman was more guarded; he famously commented when asked whether we can cure cancer, "Yes, in mice". Unfortunately, his guarded response appears to have been appropriate – initial promising results for Endostatin and other anti-angiogenesis agents have not (yet) translated into a major impact on cancer therapy.

A recent report describing an age-dependent heritable mechanism of cancer resistance in mice has suggested a possible explanation for the discrepancy between murine and human results[25].

Summary

In order to understand the molecular biology of cancer it is necessary to first obtain an understanding of normal cell biology and then to appreciate the ways in which the malignant cell subverts the normal processes.

Key elements in normal cell biology are the controls exerted over cell growth and division by internal checks, by the requirement for external growth factors, the efficacy of proofreading of DNA replication and the limit on division numbers for all non-stem cells.

The crucial elements of malignant transformation are:

- Immortality
- Independence
- Mobility
- Subversion
- Genomic Instability
- Angiogenesis induction

Cancer arises when genetic defects accumulate in the genome of a single cell which allows it to escape normal controls on growth, division and cell death. Genetic defects may occur via a variety of pathways leading to loss or gain of genetic material and/or rearrangement of material within the genome. In normal cells, highly sensitive mechanisms detect such abnormalities and induce repair or apoptosis. In tumour cells, these mechanisms are defective and cells with abnormal genomic complement can survive and give rise to malignant clones.

Understanding of the underlying mechanisms of malignant transformation is increasingly being applied to design of therapies.

References

1. Clark, D.P. & Russell, L.D. (1997) *Molecular Biology Made Simple and Fun*. Cache River Press, Vienna, Illinois.
2. Lewis, R. (ed.) (1992) *Life*. W.C. Brown, Dubuque.

3. Aerssens, J., Armstrong, M., Gilissen, R. & Cohen, N. (2001) The human genome: An introduction. *Oncologist*, **6**, 100–109.

4. Krontiris, T.G. (1995) Oncogenes: Molecular medicine. *The New England Journal of Medicine*, **333**, 303–306.

5. Boveri, T. (1914) *Zur Frage der Entstehung Maligner Tumoren* (*The Origin of Malignant Tumours*). Gustav Fisher, Jena.

6. Hahn, W.C. & Weinberg, R.A. (2002) Rules for making human tumor cells. *The New England Journal of Medicine*, **347**, 1593–1603.

7. Kerr, J.F., Wyllie, A.H. & Currie, A.R. (1972) Apoptosis: A basic biological phenomenon with wide-ranging implications in tissue kinetics. *British Journal of Cancer*, **26**, 239–257.

8. Wyllie, A.H. (1974) Death in normal and neoplastic cells. *Journal of Clinical Pathology. Supplement (Royal College of Pathologists)*, **7**, 35–42.

9. Kendall, S.D., Linardic, C.M., Adam, S.J. & Counter, C.M. (2005) A network of genetic events sufficient to convert normal cells to a tumorigenic state. *Cancer Research*, **65**, 9824–9828.

10. Campbell, K. (2000) *The Genetic Basis of Cancer*. Nursing Times, London.

11. Lakhani, S.R., Dilly, S.A. & Finlayson, C.J. (1998) Healing and repair. In: *Basic Pathology: An Introduction to the Mechanisms of Disease* (eds S.R. Lakhani, S.A. Dilly & C.J. Finlayson), pp. 78–86. Arnold, London.

12. Conover, J.C. & Notti, R.Q. (2008) The neural stem cell niche. *Cell and Tissue Research*, **331**, 211–224.

13. Campbell, K. (2002) Bone marrow as a reservoir of pluripotential stem cells for somatic growth, repair and regeneration. www.bloodmed.com. 6-9-2007.

14. Lewis, R. (1992) Mitosis. In: *Life* (ed. R. Lewis), pp. 130–151. W.C. Brown, Dubuque.

15. Hayflick, L. (1965) The limited in vitro lifetime of human diploid cell strains. *Experimental Cell Research*, **37**, 614–636.

16. Kelland, L.R. (2001) Telomerase: Biology and phase I trials. *The Lancet Oncology*, **2**, 95–102.

17. Bellon, M. & Nicot, C. (2008) Regulation of telomerase and telomeres: Human tumor viruses take control. *Journal of the National Cancer Institute*, **100**, 98–108.

18. Hoffbrand, A.V., Pettit, J.E. & Moss, P.A. (2001) The genetics of haematological malignancies. In: *Essential Haematology* (eds A.V. Hoffbrand, J.E. Pettit & P.A. Moss), pp. 145–161. Blackwell Science, Oxford.

19. Rous, P. (1911) A sarcoma of the fowl transmissible by an agent separable from the tumor cells. *The Journal of Experimental Medicine*, **XIII**, 397–411.

20. Rous, P. (1910) A transmissible avian neoplasm. (Sarcoma of the common fowl.) *The Journal of Experimental Medicine*, **12**, 696–705.

21. Franks, M. & Teich, N. M. (1997) *Introduction to the Cellular and Molecular Biology of Cancer*, Oxford Univercity Press, Oxford.

22. Knudson, A.G. (2001) Two genetic hits (more or less) to cancer. *Nature Reviews. Cancer*, **1**, 157–170.

23. Culotta, E. & Koshland, D.E.K. Jr. (1993) p53 sweeps through cancer research. *Science* **262**, 1958–1961.

24. Ide, A.G., Baker, N.H. & Warren, S.L. (1939) Vascularization of the brown Pearce rabbit epithelioma transplant as seen in the transparent ear chamber. *American Journal of Roentgenology*, **42**, 891–899.

25. Campbell, K. (2003) Of mice and men. *The Lancet Oncology*, **4**, 334.

4 Biological background

The previous chapter has given a basic outline of the biology of cancer. This chapter will address this biological background in the context of infection-associated cancer (IAC).

A seminal paper at the turn of the millennium[1] proposed that all the changes associated with carcinogenesis could be classified into six fundamental alterations in cell physiology:

- Self-sufficiency in growth signals
- Insensitivity to growth inhibitory signals
- Evasion of apoptosis
- Limitless replicative potential
- Sustained angiogenesis
- Tissue invasion and metastasis

The first four of these are relatively early stage events and are known to be induced by some infections; the last two are late events and often occur at a stage when a tumour has become autonomous – it no longer requires the infectious stimulus and cannot be cured by eradicating the infection. It is doubtful that any infection can cause *all* necessary changes. Certain infections are deemed 'necessary but not sufficient' as causes of certain cancers, but even in these cases only a small proportion of infected persons develop cancer. Additional factors are required for cancer to develop – these may be host factors such as genetic predisposition, microbial factors such as papillomavirus strain or external risk modifying factors such as smoking – all three of these have been shown to be relevant to cervical cancer development[2].

It is estimated that a normal adult body has about 10^{13} human cells but contains, mainly in the gut, about 10^{14} microbial cells – from a bacterial viewpoint we make ideal transport/culture medium, offering a protected internal milieu and plentiful nutrition. In early 2010, the journal *Nature* published a genome catalogue

Infectious Causes of Cancer, first edition. By Ken Campbell. Published 2011 by John Wiley & Sons Ltd.
© 2011 John Wiley & Sons Ltd.

for the human gut flora[3]. Given that microbes have viruses of their own, not considering those infecting our own cells, it is probably impossible to even estimate the amount of viral DNA contained by an average person's body. Persing has pointed out that '*In purely reductionist terms, infectious diseases can be viewed as horizontally acquired genetic disorders in which exogenously acquired nucleic acids of a pathogen interact chromosomally, episomally, or extracellularly with those of the host to disrupt normal cellular processes or to produce inflammation*'[4]. It is unsurprising that the disruption of host cell behaviour is capable of giving rise to malignant tumours.

Oncogenes and tumour suppressor genes

A complex network of regulatory genes controls cell division and the integrity of the genome; cells are programmed to repair errors in DNA copying, and if this fails they are programmed to self-destruct. Unregulated cell division is a threat to the whole organism so normal cells can only divide in response to an external signal – they cannot autonomously 'decide' to divide. Oncogenes drive cell growth and division, whereas tumour suppressor genes restrain this process; they are comparable to a car's accelerator and brakes. A single (rogue) oncogene can drive cell division; multiple tumour suppressor genes must fail before control is lost, just as most cars have multiple braking systems but a single accelerator.

Oncogenes are positive regulators of cell growth, initially recognized as elements of the genome of RNA tumour viruses. The common functional characteristic of oncogenes is that they drive a process required for '*tumour initiation, progression, invasion or metastasis*'[5]. Stéhelin and his colleagues reported in 1976 that the normal avian genome contains sequences related to the transforming gene(s) of avian sarcoma viruses[6]. It is now considered that the most plausible explanation is that viruses, in the process of replication, often pick up elements of the host genome, which may include host oncogenes. Oncogenes found in the genome of their origin species are called cellular oncogenes (c-onc), while those found in viral genomes are called viral oncogenes (v-onc).

Multi-stage carcinogenesis – initiation, promotion and progression

Almost all cancers develop through distinct stages – multi-stage carcinogenesis. Initiation involves DNA alterations (usually irreversible), promotion leads to transformation of initiated cells to a fully malignant phenotype, and progression (which is not seen in all cancers) leads to local invasion, angiogenesis and metastasis. Not all carcinogens are equal – there is a critical distinction between initiation and promotion.

An initiating agent induces permanent, heritable DNA damage but this is not enough for a malignant tumour to develop. A promoter drives cells which have undergone initiation to full malignant transformation. Any agent which can act as an initiator or a promoter is known as a carcinogen. Some are complete carcinogens and can act as both initiator and promoter; incomplete carcinogens can act as *either* initiator *or* promoter. Timing is critical, as promoters can only transform cells which have undergone initiation; if a cell is exposed, even repeatedly, to a tumour promoter and then to an initiator no cancer will result. Most promoters require repeated application to induce malignant transformation – in many instances one, or a few, exposures of initiated cells to promoter will induce pre-malignant lesions, but these will typically regress if the promoter is withdrawn. A threshold is reached beyond which further exposure to promoter is no longer required, and a malignant lesion will inevitably develop. An experimental model often used in the study of this process is the development of skin cancers in mice[7].

Malignant tumours eventually develop an autonomous blood supply – angiogenesis – and, in a high proportion of cases, will spread to distant sites – metastasis. Angiogenesis is necessary for a tumour to grow beyond about 2 mm. Malignant tumours produce angiogenesis-inducing factors, which are the same as those produced by normal tissues during embryological growth and tissue repair. Typically angiogenesis precedes metastasis; this is unsurprising, since highly vascular tumours shed cancer cells into the circulation at a high rate. Metastatic tumours occur only when a malignant cell embeds in a hospitable tissue environment – the 'soil and seed hypothesis'[8]. *'Several million cells per gram of tumour can be shed daily into the lymphatic system or bloodstream'*[9]; the fate of these cells is unknown, but different cancer sites are associated with different patterns of metastasis and some tissues are more prone to harbour metastases[10]. The hypothesis is that cancer cells are more likely to lodge in certain sites and, more importantly, they can only grow in sites with a hospitable microenvironment.

The main significance of the initiation, promotion and progression model is that infections contributing to carcinogenesis may act at any of these stages; EBV is thought to induce irreversible changes leading to a population of immortalized B-memory cells, cirrhosis induced by hepatitis virus infection leads to a high rate of cell division increasing the risk of hepatocellular carcinoma and *Helicobacter pylori* induces secretion of angiogenesis factors.

Key points

▪ Experimental and epidemiological evidence indicates that most tumours result from at least two exposures which may occur many years apart
▪ Certain exposures act as initiators – they cause irreversible DNA alterations
▪ Certain exposures act as promoters – they drive malignant progression in cells already altered by an initiator
▪ Promoter effects are typically reversible – they only cause tumour formation if applied repeatedly
▪ In high doses, certain exposures may act as both initiator and promoter – complete carcinogens

■ Order of exposure is critically important – initiator followed by repeated doses of promoter produces tumours, exposure to promoter followed by exposure to initiator produces no tumours

Multi-hit theory of carcinogenesis

Multi-stage carcinogenesis applies at the level of tissue exposure; the multi-hit theory applies at a cellular level. An individual cell must sustain multiple genetic abnormalities before it can undergo malignant transformation. Evidence to support this long-held theory came with Knudson's paper on retinoblastoma – a tumour of the eye seen most often in children[11]. Retinoblastoma presents in two distinct fashions;

■ Hereditary
  o Early diagnosis of first tumour
  o Often bilateral
  o May be family history
■ Sporadic
  o Later onset
  o Unilateral
  o No family history

Knudson concluded that this pattern arose because the development of a tumour required both copies of a particular gene to be inactivated in the same cell. In the familial form one defective copy was inherited and one inactivated by acquired mutation; in the sporadic form both copies were inactivated by acquired mutations. In the familial form every retinal stem cell is one mutation away from malignant transformation – it is probable that this would occur early and bilaterally. The sporadic form requires the same to acquire by chance, inactivating mutations in both copies of the same gene – likely to happen later in childhood and extremely unlikely to happen independently in both eyes.

Knudson originally referred to this new class of cancer-related gene as anti-oncogenes, although they are now known as tumour suppressor genes[12]. Tumour suppressor is more appropriate as the normal function of 'oncogenes' is to regulate cell division, while tumour suppressor genes' primary function is to inhibit inappropriate cell division, so suppressing tumour growth.

Two hits represent the minimum required for malignant transformation; most tumours have more than two mutations. It has been estimated that, by the time they are diagnosed, colon cancers may contain as many as 11 000 separate mutations[13]. *In vitro* studies[14–16] found that malignant transformation of normal human fibroblasts requires aberrant expression of at least four, possibly five, genes. Retinoblastoma arises in stem cell programmed to divide, hence the only change needed is loss of tumour suppression by the Rb protein. The requirement for multiple independent events accounts for the long delay commonly seen between infection and development of overt malignancy – in the case of hepatocellular carcinoma this may be as much as 50 years[17].

Direct and indirect carcinogenesis

Direct carcinogenic exposures alter individual cells increasing the risk of malignant transformation; indirect carcinogens act at tissue level to increase the risk of emergence of a malignant clone. Initiators, which induce irreversible DNA changes, are direct carcinogens, whereas many promoters are indirect carcinogens. In many instances promoters are thought to act by increasing the cell turnover – by increasing the population dividing this increases the risk of a cell acquiring a second mutation. A classic setting for this is inflammation and Virchow recognized the link between inflammation and cancer in the late nineteenth century[18]. There are several forms of IAC in which inflammation is a key pathway in oncogenesis; these include H. pylori and stomach cancer and hepatitis viruses and hepatocellular carcinoma (HCC). HCC is particularly striking, in that the consequence of primary viral infection depends to a large extent on the immune status of the host. Infection of an immunocompetent adult typically leads to an acute infection, often asymptomatic, followed in 95% of cases by clearance of the virus; infants (or others with reduced immunity) have a high probability of being chronically infected, which in a proportion of cases will lead to cirrhosis and possibly hepatocellular carcinoma[19, 20].

Infections may trigger cancer either directly by transforming cells or indirectly, by creating conditions under which malignant transformation is more likely to occur[21]. Certain infections act as direct carcinogens; they encode oncoproteins which may dysregulate cell cycle, affect the telomere/telomerase system or alter apoptotic or other cell pathways – these include HPV, EBV, HTLV-1 and HHV8. There are other infections, such as HBV, HCV, H. pylori which act indirectly by inducing chronic inflammation with a necrotic and proliferative response, favouring emergence of malignant clones. HIV appears to represent a different form of indirect carcinogenesis; it suppresses the immune system and thus increases the incidence of other tumorigenic infections.

Inflammation and cancer

Evidence that chronic irritation and inflammation can be carcinogenic is given by the association between drinking of scalding hot beverages, such as Maté tea in South America, and oesophageal cancer[22]; the extremely hot beverages cause mucosal damage, cells divide rapidly in the process of tissue repair and this creates a background in which oncogenesis is more likely to occur. There are many other known risk factors for oesophageal cancer; tobacco and excess alcohol[23] are definite risk factors and some reports indicate that papillomavirus infection may also contribute[24]. Inflammation alone is insufficient to induce malignant disease;

it creates a population of cells which are particularly vulnerable to other carcinogenic exposures. A situation, in which an area of epithelium undergoes changes which may predispose to development of cancer, is known as *field cancerization*[25].

In many cases of infection-associated cancer field carcinogenesis, secondary to chronic inflammation, is a key mechanism. Evidence in support of this is supplied by the behaviour of MALT-lymphomas, in which the early stage of malignant transformation appears to be driven by *H. pylori* infection and treatment of the infection can lead to resolution of the lymphoma[26]; at a later stage, following acquisition of further genetic alterations, the lymphoma no longer requires *H. pylori* as a driver and infection eradication is unlikely to lead to lymphoma resolution[27].

Latency and penetrance

In some forms of carcinogenesis, there may be a lag of many years, even decades, between initial exposure and diagnosis of cancer – latency. This is a common phenomenon in IAC; it is commonly associated with a very low percentage of infected persons developing cancer – low penetrance.

The time of infection with HTLV-1 can often be precisely determined and typically precedes diagnosis of associated Adult T-cell leukaemia/lymphoma by many years: in Japan the typical latency is about 60 years[28], and only about 6% of males and 2% of females who carry HTLV-1 will go on to develop adult T-cell leukemia/lymphoma (ATL)[29].

Both of these aspects are consistent with induction of a population of premalignant cells by the infection, followed by random mutations within that population. A cancer arises only when a particular cell hits the malevolent 'jackpot' and acquires the full repertoire of gene changes required for malignant transformation. Whether one adopts the traditional 'serial' model, in which these changes are acquired stepwise with emergence of successive clones each containing more cancer-predisposing mutations, or the new 'parallel' model, in which all of the changes occur in cells of one of many clones existing at the same time, it will take many generations on average for a malignancy to emerge. The need for multiple complementary mutations to occur in the same clone, by whichever mechanism, also explains the low rate of transformation of pre-malignant lesions to frank malignancies.

Specific mechanisms of carcinogenesis relevant to infection-associated cancer (IAC)

Viruses, unsurprisingly, are more common causes of cancer than bacteria or parasites. A virus is a mobile package of genetic information – to survive and multiply it will exploit or control the host cell's pathways for cell growth, division and apoptosis – to escape the immune system it will induce immunosuppression or deploy 'stealth technology' to hide the host cell from the immune system; any of these taken alone increases the risk of the emergence of a malignant population, taken together the danger is clear.

Typically, viral infections associated with cancers establish latent infections or persistent sub-clinical infections, which are long-term infections in which there is no overt disease – the virus 'lies low' within its host. Lytic infections, in which there is rapid production of virus particles which burst (lyse) the host cell, tend to cause acute illnesses and are eradicated by the host immune system. The formal definition of viral latency is that viral DNA is present in host cells but there is no replication and no release of new virus particles. The viral genetic material may be integrated into the host genome or it may be free within the cell, in a form known as an episome. In persistent viral infection there is low-level viral replication and infection of new cells within the host but without triggering clinical signs or symptoms.

True latency occurs in cells with extremely low turnover, such as neurons (e.g. Herpes simplex) or memory B-cells (e.g. EBV). In these tissues there is little expression of viral RNA or protein and hence little risk of triggering an immune response. There is commonly an initial cytocidal phase of the infection – this may be accompanied by a brief flu-like illness; in other cases the initial infectious phase is entirely sub-clinical. It is probable that the clinically overt phase, when it occurs, reflects the immune response and clearance of the virus population from dividing cells; this leaves latent infection present in non-dividing cells.

In some cases there is a low-level war of attrition between the virus and the immune system. Varicella-zoster latent infection of dorsal root ganglia of the spine may follow chicken pox; latency persists in such cases for decades. When a host becomes immunodeficient (e.g. cancer or its treatment, old age), the virus may spread along the nerve trunks and cause shingles. There is no evidence that an active trigger is required – loss of adequate immune surveillance is all that is needed for the virus to emerge from quiescence and cause a painful and disabling disease.

For several tumour types the presence of lymphocytes within the tumour mass, 'tumour-infiltrating lymphocytes – TIL', is a significant prognostic factor[30]. This had been foreshadowed by a report almost a century earlier of the key role of lymphocytes in cancer immunity[31]. This phenomenon is not confined to infection-associated malignancies, indeed it was first reported in melanoma. A detailed discussion of cancer immunology is beyond the scope of this text; this area has been discussed in several excellent recent reviews[32–34].

Chronic persistent infection may occur in more active tissues provided that the virus is only minimally cytotoxic. As previously commented, hepatitis viruses cause little direct damage to the liver; the immune response leads to inflammation, followed by cirrhosis and, potentially, hepatocellular carcinoma (HCC). A strong immune response eradicates infection rapidly with minimal or no long-term sequelae; a weak response leads to a modus vivendi in which the immune system will let the virus be as long as damage is minimal[35]. The problem arises when the immune response is sufficient to damage liver cells but not brisk enough to eradicate infection. In this case the condition chronic active hepatitis (CAH) ensues, which leads to progressive liver damage, cirrhosis and HCC. Referring to a transgenic murine model, Chisari remarks, *'the results suggest that an ineffective immune response is the principal oncogenic factor during chronic HBV infection in man. It is ironic that the same T cell response that can eradicate HBV from the liver when it is strong can be procarcinogenic by triggering a chronic necroinflammatory liver disease when it is unable to completely terminate the infection'*[36].

Integration of viral genetic material into genome

One mechanism of viral oncogenesis is insertion of a viral oncogene into the genome of a host cell; this will only lead to malignant transformation if expression of the oncogene is triggered by a positive regulatory signal. The worst case scenario is that an oncogene is inserted in a position normally occupied by a constitutively expressed gene; this will ensure that a gene which is normally very closely regulated is instead continuously expressed, driving forward the processes of cell growth and division. [A constitutively expressed gene is one which is expressed as part of the normal functioning of the cell – they are sometimes also called 'household' genes reflecting their status as functions expressed in all cells at a low level.] Alternatively, a positive regulatory sequence may be inserted in a position in which it will promote expression of a cellular oncogene. Tumour suppressor genes may be prevented from exerting their normal braking effects by insertion of a negative regulatory sequence upstream of the suppressor. In either case, this process is known as 'insertional mutagenesis'.

Presence of viral DNA/RNA in malignant cell but outwith cell genome

All cells contain sequences of DNA outwith the chromosomes; the most prevalent example of this is mitochondrial DNA (mtDNA), which is found only in the cytoplasm, contained within mitochondria. Almost 100% of mtDNA is maternally derived; although some paternal mitochondria are transferred to the ovum at fertilization, these are eliminated rapidly and failure of this process may impair normal embryonic development[37]. Mitochondria are believed to be free-living organisms which became endosymbionts of eukaryotic cells[38].

A number of viruses with carcinogenic potential establish a latent infection on first entering host cells; this is frequently associated with the presence of episomal virus DNA. [An episome is a *'unit of genetic material that is composed of a series of genes that sometimes has an independent existence in a host cell and at other times is integrated into a chromosome of the cell, replicating itself along with the chromosome'*[38].] An episome may be present as a sequence integrated within the host genome, or as extrachromosomal DNA, typically in the form of a loop. Episomal DNA is copied when the cell divides and is present in each daughter cell, thus maintaining a low-level infection without provoking an immune response of the type caused by lytic infection. A single virus may produce both types of episome, for example HPV is primarily extrachromosomal in early stages and is integrated into host chromosomes in invasive lesions[39]. Initial infection of the uterine cervix by HPV probably occurs in the stem cells of the basal epithelium; HPV genomes are established as extrachromosomal elements, known as episomes, within the cytoplasm[38]. In invasive cervical cancer parts of the HPV genome are integrated into the host cell genome; the sites of integration are variable between individuals but unique in any one patient, which confirms the clonal nature of the tumour cells[40]. Integration of viral DNA does not consistently involve sites in which insertional mutagenesis is likely; it does involve loss of regulatory sequences which normally restrict expression of viral oncogenes[41].

Causation versus association

One of the difficulties in determining whether an organism is causally associated with a specific cancer is *confounding*; this refers to a statistically significant correlation between two factors where there is no causal association. An example would be greater prevalence of a particular disease in married women, in some cases such an association may be real but there is great potential for confounding. The most obvious confounding element in this case is age – many diseases become more common with increasing age and older women are statistically more likely to be married than younger ones. The easiest way to demonstrate the possibility of such a confounder effect is to look at the age profiles of the populations being compared – if they differ markedly, the relationship is only likely to be relevant if it is known that the disease of interest has an age-independent distribution. Griffiths has pointed out that it is probable that such confounding explains, to a large part, the observation that cervical cancer is more common in married women than in single women[42].

In some cases it is possible to demonstrate with confidence that a given factor is more likely to be a confounder than a true causal agent; in other cases the relationship is more complex and it may be difficult to differentiate between confounders and cofactors. An example, which took many years to resolve, is the role of Herpes Simplex Virus (HSV) as a causative agent for cervical cancer. Ramazzini, the father of occupational medicine, had observed in the eighteenth century that the pattern of breast and uterine cancer in nuns differed from that in the laity[43]. The following century Rigoni-Stern published similar observations comparing nuns to married women, he makes no mention of Ramazzini's prior work[44]; By the 1960s, over a century after Rigoni-Stern's paper, it was speculated that a transmissible agent was responsible for the disease, and that this might be genital HSV (HSV2)[45]. Plausible serological evidence[46] and an animal model supported the hypothesis[47].

Accumulated evidence gradually led away from HSV and towards Human Papillomavirus (HPV) as an infective cause of cervical cancer[48]. It is now accepted that HPV infection is a necessary but not sufficient cause of cervical cancer, while HSV infection is one of several factors which increase the risk[49]. The high seroprevalence in early studies is unsurprising given that, in a study[50] of Korean sex workers the incidence of HPV positivity was found to be 83.5% and that for HSV2 86.2% – clearly many of the subjects would have tested positive for both viruses.

The distinction is vital – a vaccine is now being introduced against the strains of HPV most associated with the risk of cervical cancer; it has been estimated that this has the potential to reduce the number of high-grade pre-cancerous lesions by 66% and cervical cancer deaths by 76% in the UK[51]. The impact of a vaccine against HSV2 would be minimal since this is not a necessary cause of cervical cancer and there are other cofactors.

A recent paper has proposed that *Helicobacter* species may be cofactors to hepatitis C virus infection in causation of hepatocellular carcinoma[52]. Here again, the primary evidence is finding of *Helicobacter* species in diseased liver; the question which must be answered is whether this is coincidental – mere association – or causal.

Transmissible tumours

There are no known human transmissible tumours. The best characterized instance of a transmissible tumour occurs in dogs – canine transmissible venereal tumour (CTVT), all known examples of which are genetically identical[53]. CTVT has been recognized as a tumour type for over 130 years[54], while in his 1910 paper on a transmissible avian tumour Rous makes reference to '*a sarcoma of the dog, transmissible at coitus*'[55]. The accepted mechanism of spread of CTVT is transfer of malignant cells during sexual contact[53]. The tumour becomes established in the host but does not metastasize in mature animals and typically regresses and disappears within about 3–4 months. Although the tumour clearly evades immune surveillance during the phase of invasion and consolidation, an animal which has once been 'infected' by the tumour mounts an effective immune response on re-challenge. CTVT rarely causes death; it establishes itself, persists for long enough to have a high probability of sexual transfer and then regresses.

Evidence suggests that the facial-tumour disease which afflicts Tasmanian Devils in the wild may also be a transmissible tumour[56], although other authors believe this to be due to an, as yet uncharacterized, virus.

References

1. Hanahan, D. & Weinberg, R.A. (2000) The hallmarks of cancer. *Cell*, **100**, 57–70.

2. Bosch, F.X. & Iftner, T. (2005) *The Aetiology of Cervical Cancer*. NHS Cancer Screening Programmes, Sheffield.

3. Li, R., Qin, J., Raes, J., Arumugam, M., Burgdorf, K.S., Manichanh, C., Nielsen, T., Pons, N., Levenez, F., Yamada, T., Mende, D.R., Li, J., Xu, J., Li, S., Li, D., Cao, J., Wang, B., Liang, H., Zheng, H., Xie, Y., Tap, J., Lepage, P., Bertalan, M., Batto, J-M., Hansen, T., Le Paslier, D., Linneberg, A., Nielsen, H.B., Pelletier, E., Renault, P., Sicheritz-Ponten, T., Turner, K., Zhu, H., Yu, C., Li, S., Jian, M., Zhou, Y., Li, Y., Zhang, X., Li, S., Qin, N., Yang, H., Wang, J., Brunak, S., Dore, J, Guarner, F., Kristiansen, K., Pedersen, O., Parkhill, J., Weissenbach, J., MetaHIT Consortium, Bork, P., Ehrlich, S.D. & Wang, J. (2010) A human gut microbial gene catalogue established by metagenomic sequencing. *Nature*, **464**, 59–67.

4. Persing, D.H. & Prendergast, F.G. (1999) Infection, immunity, and cancer. *Archives of Pathology & Laboratory Medicine*, **123**, 1015–1022.

5. Boyle, P. & Levin, B. (2008) Genetic susceptibility. In: *World Cancer Report 2008* (eds. P. Boyle & B. Levin), Chap. 2.15, pp. 182–185. International Agency for Research on Cancer, Lyon.

6. Stéhelin, D., Varmus, H.E., Bishop, J.M. & Vogt, P.K. (1976) DNA related to the transforming gene(s) of avian sarcoma viruses is present in normal avian DNA. *Nature*, **260**, 170–173.

7. Perez-Losada, J. & Balmain, A. (2003) Stem-cell hierarchy in skin cancer. *Nature Reviews. Cancer*, **3**, 436–443.

8. Paget, S. (1889) The distribution of secondary growths in cancer of the breast. *Lancet*, **1**, 571–573.

9. Butler, T.P. & Gullino, P.M. (1975) Quantitation of cell shedding into efferent blood of mammary adenocarcinoma. *Cancer Research*, **35**, 512–516.

10. Fidler, I.J. (2003) The pathogenesis of cancer metastasis: The 'seed and soil' hypothesis revisited. *Nature Reviews. Cancer*, **3**, 453–458.

11. Knudson, A.G. Jr. (1971) Mutation and cancer: Statistical study of retinoblastoma. *Proceedings of the National Academy of Sciences of the United States of America*, **68**, 820–823.

12. Knudson, A.G. (2001) Two genetic hits (more or less) to cancer. *Nature Reviews. Cancer*, **1**, 157–162.

13. Stoler, D.L., Chen, N., Basik, M., Kahlenberg, M.S., Rodriguez-Bigas, M.A., Petrelli, N.J. & Anderson, G.R. (1999) The onset and extent of genomic instability in sporadic colorectal tumor progression. *Proceedings of the National Academy of Sciences of the United States of America*, **96**, 15121–15126.

14. Hahn, W.C., Counter, C.M., Lundberg, A.S., Beijersbergen, R.L., Brooks, M.W. & Weinberg, R.A. (1999) Creation of human tumour cells with defined genetic elements. *Nature*, **400**, 464–468.

15. Hahn, W.C. & Weinberg, R.A. (2002) Rules for making human tumor cells. *The New England Journal of Medicine*, **347**, 1594–1603.

16. Kendall, S.D., Linardic, C.M., Adam, S.J. & Counter, C.M. (2005) A network of genetic events sufficient to convert normal human cells to a tumorigenic state. *Cancer Research*, **65**, 9824–9828.

17. Schottenfeld, D. & Beebe-Dimmer, J. (2006) Chronic inflammation: A common and important factor in the pathogenesis of neoplasia. *CA: A Cancer Journal for Clinicians*, **56**, 69–83.

18. Virchow, R. (1858) Die Cellularpathologie in ihrer Begründung auf physiologische und pathologische Gewebelehre (*Cellular Pathology as Based upon Physiological and Pathological Histology*). A. Hirschwald, Berlin.

19. Goldstein, S.T., Zhou, F., Hadler, S.C., Bell, B.P., Mast, E.E. & Margolis, H.S. (2005) A mathematical model to estimate global hepatitis B disease burden and vaccination impact. *International Journal of Epidemiology*, **34**, 1329–1339.

20. Lupberger, J. & Hildt, E. (2007) Hepatitis B virus-induced oncogenesis. *World Journal of Gastroenterology*, **13**, 74–81.

21. Boyle, P. & Levin, B. (2008) Chronic infections. In: *World Cancer Report 2008* (eds. P. Boyle & B. Levin), Chap. 2.5, pp. 128–135. International Agency for Research on Cancer, Lyon.

22. De Stefani, E., Muñoz, N., Esteve, J., Vasallo, A., Victora, C.G. & Teuchmann, S. (1990) Maté drinking, alcohol, tobacco, diet, and esophageal cancer in Uruguay. *Cancer Research*, **50**, 426–431.

23. Wood, H., Brewster, D. & Møller, H. (2005) Oesophagus. In: *Cancer Altlas of the United Kingdom and Ireland 1991–2001* (eds. M. Quinn, H. Wood, N. Copper & S. Rowar), Chap. 17, pp. 183–192. Palgrave Macmillan, Basingstoke.

24. de Villiers, E.M., Lavergne, D., Chang, F., Syrjanen, K., Tosi, P., Cinrotino, M., Santopietro, R. & Syrganen, S. (1999) An interlaboratory study to determine the presence of human papillomavirus DNA in esophageal carcinoma from China. *International Journal of Cancer*, **81**, 225–228.

25. Dakubo, G.D., Jakupciak, J.P., Birch-Machin, M.A. & Parr, R.L. (2007) Clinical implications and utility of field cancerization. *Cancer Cell International*, **7**, 2.

26. Wotherspoon, A.C., Doglioni, C., Diss, T.C., Pan, L., Moschini, A., De Boni, M. & Isaacson, P.G. (1993) Regression of primary low-grade B-cell gastric lymphoma of mucosa-associated lymphoid tissue type after eradication of *Helicobacter pylori*. *Lancet*, **342**, 575–577.

27. Wotherspoon, A.C. (2000) A critical review of the effect of *Helicobacter pylori* eradication on gastric MALT lymphoma. *Current Gastroenterology Reports*, **2**, 494–498.

28. Takatsuki, K., Yamaguchi, K. & Matsuoka, M. (1994) ATL and HTLV-1-related diseases. In: *Adult T-cell Leukemia* (eds. K. Tabatsubi), Chap. 1, pp. 1–27. Oxford University Press, Oxford.

29. Arisawa, K., Soda, M., Endo, S. et al. (2000) Evaluation of adult T-cell leukemia/lymphoma incidence and its impact on non-Hodgkin lymphoma incidence in southwestern Japan. *International Journal of Cancer*, **85**, 319–324.

30. Swann, J.B. & Smyth, M.J. (2007) Immune surveillance of tumors. *The Journal of Clinical Investigation*, **117**, 1137–1146.

31. Murphy, J.B. & Morton, J.J. (1915) The lymphocyte as a factor in natural and induced resistance to transplanted cancer. *Proceedings of the National Academy of Sciences of the United States of America*, **1**, 435–437.

32. Baron, F. & Storb, R. (2006) The immune system as a foundation for immunologic therapy and hematologic malignancies: A historical perspective. *Best Practice & Research Clinical Haematology*, **19**, 637–653.

33. Mantovani, A., Romero, P., Palucka, A.K. & Marincola, F.M. (2008) Tumour immunity: Effector response to tumour and role of the microenvironment. *Lancet*, **371**, 771–783.

34. Prestwich, R.J., Errington, F., Hatfield, P., Merrick, A.E., Ilett, E.J., Selby, P.J. & Melcher, A.A. (2008) The immune system – Is it relevant to cancer development, progression and treatment? *Clinical Oncology*, **20**, 101–112.

35. Chwla, Y. (2005) Hepatitis B virus: Inactive carriers. *Virology Journal*, **2**, 82.

36. Chisari, F.V. (2000) Viruses, immunity and cancer: Lessons from hepatitis B. *The American Journal of Pathology*, **156**, 1118–1132.

37. Krawetz, S.A. (2005) Paternal contribution: New insights and future challenges. *Nature Reviews Genetics*, **6**, 633–642.

38. Tinnis, J.N., Ayliffe, M.A., Huang, C.Y.& Martin, W. (2004) Endosymbiotic gene transfer: Organelle genomes forge eukaryotic chromosomes. *Nature Reviews Genetics*, **5**, 123–135.

39. Hudelist, G., Manavi, M., Pischinger, K.I., Watkins-Riedel, T., Singer, C.F., Kubista, E. & Czerwenka, K.F. (2004) Physical state and expression of HPV DNA in benign and dysplastic cervical tissue: Different levels of viral integration are correlated with lesion grade. *Gynecologic Oncology*, **92**, 873–880.

40. Woodman, C.B., Collins, S.I. & Young, L.S. (2007) The natural history of cervical HPV infection: Unresolved issues. *Nature Reviews Cancer*, **7**, 11–22.

41. Choo, K.B., Pan, C.C. & Han, S.H. (1987) Integration of human papillomavirus type 16 into cellular DNA of cervical carcinoma: Preferential deletion of the E2 gene and invariable retention of the long control region and the E6/E7 open reading frames. *Virology*, **161**, 259–261.

42. Griffiths, M. (1991) 'Nuns, virgins, and spinsters'. Rigoni-Stern and cervical cancer revisited. *British Journal of Obstetrics and Gynaecology*, **98**, 797–802.

43. Ramazzini, B. (1940) De morbis artificum (*Diseases of Workers*-translation by Wilmer Cave Wright). University of Chicago Press, Chicago.

44. Rigorni-Stern, D.A. (1987) Fatti statistici relativi alle malattic cancerose…(Statistical facts about cancers on which Doctor Rigoni-Stern based his contribution to the Surgeons' Subgroup of the

IV Congress of the Italian Scientists on 23 September 1842 – Translation of Classical Article). *Statistics in Medicine*, **6**, 881–884.

45. Rawls, W.E., Tompkins, W.A., Figueroa, M.E. & Melnick, J.L. (1968) Herpesvirus type 2: Association with carcinoma of the cervix. *Science*, **161**, 255–256.

46. Koenig, U.D., Haag, A. & Lehmk (1975) [Seroepidemiological studies related to the association of genital herpes to cervical cancer (author's transl)]. *Geburtshilfe Frauenheilkd*, **35**, 909–913.

47. Wentz, W.B., Reagan, J.W. & Heggie, A.D. (1975) Cervical carcinogenesis with herpes simplex virus, type 2. *Obstetrics & Gynecology*, **46**, 117–121.

48. Kitchener, H.C. (1988) Genital virus infection and cervical neoplasia. *British Journal of Obstetrics and Gynaecology*, **95**, 182–191.

49. Castellsague, X., Diaz, M., de Sanjose, S., Munoz, N., Herrero, R., Franceschi, S., Peeling, R.W., Ashley, R., Smith, J.S., Snijders, P.J., Meijer, C.J. & Bosch, F.X. (2006) Worldwide human papillomavirus etiology of cervical adenocarcinoma and its cofactors: Implications for screening and prevention. *Journal of the National Cancer Institute*, **98**, 303–315.

50. Yun, H., Park, J., Choi, I., Kee, M., Choi, B. & Kim, S. (2008) Prevalence of human papillomavirus and herpes simplex virus type 2 infection in Korean commercial sex workers. *Journal of Microbiology and Biotechnology*, **18**, 350–354.

51. Kohli, M., Ferko, N., Martin, A., Franco, E.L., Jenkins, D., Gallivan, S., Sherlaw-Johnson, C. & Drummond, M. (2007) Estimating the long-term impact of a prophylactic human papillomavirus 16/18 vaccine on the burden of cervical cancer in the UK. *British Journal of Cancer*, **96**, 143–150.

52. Pellicano, R., Menard, A., Rizzetto, M. & Megraud, F. (2008) *Helicobacter* species and liver diseases: Association or causation? *The Lancet Infectious Diseases*, **8**, 254–260.

53. Murgia, C., Pritchard, J.K., Kim, S.Y., Fassati, A. & Weiss, R.A. (2006) Clonal origin and evolution of a transmissible cancer. *Cell*, **126**, 477–487.

54. Novinski, M.A. (1876) Zur Frage uber die Impfung der Krebsigen Geschwulste. *Zentralblatt fur Medizinische Wissenschaften*, **14**, 790–791.

55. Rous, P. (1910) A transmissible avian neoplasm. (Sarcoma of the common fowl). *Journal of Experimental Medicine*, **12**, 696–705.

56. Pearse, A.M. & Swift, K. (2006) Allograft theory: Transmission of devil facial-tumour disease. *Nature*, **439**, 549.

5 Public health considerations and prevention

Infection-associated cancers typically have a very long latency between infection and diagnosis of malignancy, with a low rate of malignant transformation; the associated cancer burden is high because of the very high incidence of many of the infections. In most cases there is no way to reduce the rate of malignant transformation, so efforts to reduce the cancer rate must focus on the infectious disease.

Prevention may be divided into primary, meaning measures to prevent populations from becoming infected, and secondary, meaning interventions designed to block the clinical consequences of infection. Primary prevention depends on either blocking transmission or enhancing host immunity to prevent infection becoming established. Secondary prevention depends on interrupting the process(es) leading from infection to malignant transformation. For primary prevention a clear understanding of the route of transmission is vital, for secondary prevention it is equally necessary to have a full understanding of the pathways leading to malignant transformation.

Early primary prevention is achieved by preventing exposure to the pathogen; in the case of some parasites this may be achieved by interrupting the life cycle of the intermediate host(s). Classic primary prevention seeks to prevent establishment of infection in exposed individuals, for example measures to enhance host resistance such as vaccination. Secondary prevention may be achieved by early detection and effective treatment of the infection (schistosomiasis and bladder cancer) by reducing the level of exposure to cofactors (aflatoxins and liver cancer) or by screening for early malignant changes to allow intervention (cervical cancer).

A 2003 survey of UK cancer funding[1] reported the following breakdown of spending:

- Biology   41%
- Treatment 22%
- Aetiology 16%

Infectious Causes of Cancer, first edition. By Ken Campbell. Published 2011 by John Wiley & Sons Ltd.
© 2011 John Wiley & Sons Ltd.

- Early detection, diagnosis and prognosis   8%
- Control, survival and outcomes   6%
- Scientific model systems   5%
- Prevention   2%

The way in which the independent newspaper reports this survey is interesting, 'Critics have attacked the cancer research establishment in the past for promising much and delivering little. The research map published yesterday shows that the largest slice of funding is still being spent on biological research (41%), understanding the basic mechanisms of cancer, rather than developing new treatments (22%), or means of preventing it (2%)'[2]. The Cancer Reform Strategy (CRS) sets *'preventing cancer'* as the first of its specific objectives stating *'Over half of all cancers could be prevented by changes to lifestyle'*[3]. Unfortunately, the evidence suggests that many, perhaps most, people are unwilling to forgo cancer-risk behaviours: they continue to smoke, drink to excess, copulate indiscriminately, eat unwisely, bake in the sun, and avoid exercise. A number of the cancers associated with infection offer the possibility of protection by vaccination, a strategy which is attractive because it does not require a continuing commitment on the part of the individual.

Any attempt at primary prevention must consider the routes of transmission of relevant infections, to determine where it is feasible to block transmission. In cases where this is infeasible, for example many perinatally acquired infections, vaccination programmes are more likely to prove effective.

There are a limited number of mechanisms by which infectious diseases are spread. Traditionally it was taught that infectious diseases were spread by the 'five Fs';

- Food (and water)
- Faeces
- Flies (and other invertebrate vectors)
- Fomites (contaminated objects)
- Fornication

This list today can be seen to be incomplete, with a number of significant Fs missing. A major one is Family – it is increasingly realized that intimate, non-sexual, contact within the family environment may be implicated in the spread of both bacteria (*Helicobacter pylori*) and viruses (Epstein–Barr virus, EBV). One might stretch the F theme to accommodate Foetal micro-transfusion with maternal blood, which appears to play a part in certain viral infections – most non-viral infectious agents cannot cross the placental barrier. A very important missing F is (body) Fluids – especially the blood-borne viruses (BBV) – HIV, HBV, HCV, HTLV-1 and KSHV. Although described as blood-borne, several of these agents are also present in other bodily secretions including semen, vaginal secretions[4] and breast-milk. At one time blood transfusion was a common route of spread for BBV but the effectiveness of donor screening and testing of donated units has now reduced this to a minimal level.

The principal mode of spread of an infection may vary across different time periods; as one mode of transmission is effectively blocked it may become necessary to redefine priorities – an example of this is Hepatitis C, for which transfusion has become of negligible importance while the relative contribution of injecting drug use has risen greatly.

Routes of spread

Vertical

Vertical transmission may be prenatal, perinatal or postnatal. In the case of HIV, there is evidence that micro-transfusions from mother to infant occur during late pregnancy, and that these may lead to viral transfer[5]. Clearly, any blood-borne virus may be transferred from mother to infant during delivery; some viruses, including adult T lymphotropic virus (ATLV-1) and HIV, are present in breast-milk, and are transmitted by breast-feeding. In developed countries, where formula-feeding carries low infection risks, campaigns to reduce breast-feeding in endemic areas have dramatically lowered vertical transmission of some organisms[6].

Intrafamilial spread

Intrafamilial spread may occur in any population but is commonest in the developing world and in socio-economically deprived groups; populations often characterized by larger family sizes, cramped accommodation and lower standards of domestic and public hygiene. Spread may be faecal-oral, oral-oral, respiratory, by fomites or by blood contamination. *H. pylori* is often transmitted in this way – the risk of infection is heavily influenced by the presence of infected siblings within the same household[7].

The timing of infectious exposure can dramatically influence the clinical outcome. If a child is infected perinatally with hepatitis B, there is less than 10% chance of symptomatic disease but chronic hepatitis is very likely to ensue, potentially leading to cirrhosis and, in some cases, to hepatocellular carcinoma. Up to half of all adult acquired infection is symptomatic yet rarely has chronic sequelae. Globally, the most common route of infection is vertically, during childbirth, although this is rare in the developed world[8]. Perinatal transmission can be blocked by early vaccination of children born to HBV-positive mothers. Childhood acquired infection follows an intermediate path, still with a significant proportion remaining asymptomatic and developing chronic disease. A review of the natural history of hepatitis B is available on the web at www.mayoclinicproceedings.com[9].

For Epstein–Barr virus (EBV) the case appears to be the reverse – early, probably family-acquired, infection is asymptomatic or associated with a mild flu-like illness; late infection, in contrast, may lead to infectious mononucleosis or, rarely, to lymphoma or other cancers. Early infection with EBV may be carcinogenic if certain cofactors present in later life cause relative immunoparesis, as this may permit development of Burkitt's lymphoma.

In some instances there are distinct modes of transmission in the developing and developed worlds; and within different social groups in the latter. An example is Epstein–Barr virus – in the developing world and lower socio-economic groups in the developed world, this appears to be acquired very early in life and in almost all cases without overt clinical signs[10]. In almost all cases, primary Epstein–Barr virus is thought to be transmitted in saliva, which contains the virus for some weeks after primary infection – the long-term reservoir of virus within the body is in memory B cells, which are very unlikely to be transferred to a new host.

Intimate contact other than sexual intercourse

Some infections appear to be transmitted by non-sexual social contacts, outside the family. Epstein–Barr virus is present in saliva for weeks after primary infection and, in those who have not been infected in early childhood is thought to be acquired by intense kissing[11]. When initial infection is delayed a mild pyrexial illness may ensue – glandular fever/infectious mononucleosis[12]; this is usually self-limiting.

Sexual transmission

Unprotected sexual intercourse, vaginal, oral or anal, may lead to infection with organisms which are present in semen or in vaginal fluids. Transmission from males to females occurs with a much higher frequency, probably because of the large volume of fluid transfer with male ejaculation. It is clear that this is not, however, a necessity for infection to occur. There is clear evidence of sexual transmission of infection between lesbian couples, possibly by sharing of sex toys[13]; unfortunately, many lesbian women believe risks of female-to-female transmission are minimal or nonexistent which may encourage high-risk behaviours and discourage Pap screening[14].

Men who have sex with men are a particularly high-risk group for sexual transmission of infections; this probably relates to the frequency in this group of anal intercourse, multiple sexual partners and of multiple infections (leading to relative immunosuppression, even in HIV negative men) – this hypothesis is supported by the higher incidence of Kaposi sarcoma in HIV positive gay men than in other HIV positive groups[15]. Recent reports indicate an increasing prevalence of unprotected anal intercourse (UAI), sometimes referred to as 'bare-backing', amongst gay men in London[16]; others suggest that this practice is no longer increasing[17].

In some viral infections sexual transmission is the primary route, although it should be stressed that this is not the only route. High-risk strains of HPV are implicated in both cervical cancer and oral cancer; infection is usually acquired sexually but there are childhood cases in which transmission is believed to be by non-sexual contact[18] – this is supported by the fact that condoms do not entirely protect against infection[19], indicating transmission by skin–skin contact rather than via mucous membranes. The fact that 'heavy petting' falling short of sexual intercourse may be sufficient for transmission of the virus[20] strongly favours early, rather than late, vaccination. It is important to stress in health education that, although condoms do not completely protect against HPV, they do significantly reduce the risk and they protect against cervical cancer even where infection occurs[21] – possibly by preventing transmission of other infections, such as *Chlamydia trachomatis*, HSV-2 and HIV, which may act as cofactors[22]. They do offer very substantial protection against unwanted pregnancy and a number of other sexually-transmissible infections[23]; no mechanical barrier is 100% effective and having multiple sexual partners is a major risk factor for STIs, even with consistent condom use.

Hepatitis B virus is present in semen, saliva and blood, whereas hepatitis C virus is only present in blood of infected individuals. In the developed world the two primary routes of hepatitis B transmission are intravenous drug abuse and unprotected sex[24]. HBV is transmitted efficiently by sexual contact among heterosexuals and among men who have sex with men (MSM)[25]. Female partners of men who have sex with both men and women may be unaware that they are being placed at high risk. It has been reported by CDC that about 20% of hepatitis C transmission in the community is sexual; a more recent review has challenged the view that hepatitis C can be sexually transmitted and suggested that incidents of apparent sexual transmission result from blood transfer via contaminated objects such as razor blades and toothbrushes[26]. This is of academic, rather than practical, significance, since it is known that infection with hepatitis C may serologically mask hepatitis B infection[27]; HBV is definitely sexually transmitted, so in any case where one member of a couple is HCV positive they would be strongly advised to practice safe sex. Hepatitis D appears to be spread sexually and by blood contact in low-prevalence countries (including the UK); its mode of spread in high-prevalence areas is unknown. Measures protecting against HBV transfer are likely to also protect against HDV. Hepatitis D may be acquired at the same time as HBV – co-infection – or separately, at a later time – super-infection[28]. There is little or no incentive to develop specific prevention or vaccination programmes as its incidence inevitably declines in step with reduction in HBV incidence[29].

A major problem in reducing sexual transmission of viral infections is the refusal of the UK Prison Service to follow proven recommendations for risk reduction; this has been discussed in detail in a report published in 2005[30]. Despite many reviews and recommendations the agency has consistently refused to provide easy access to condoms within male prisons; the justification for this policy is that all sexual contact between prisons is illegal. Facultative homosexuality is common in prisons – some men, if placed in an exclusively male environment, will engage in homosexual acts which they would otherwise not contemplate, regarding themselves as entirely heterosexual[31]. Men who engage in such behaviour may, on their release, spread acquired infection widely within the heterosexual community. Although adult-acquired HBV is unlikely to lead to cancer, there is a risk that prison-acquired infection will be transmitted to sexual partners and thence, perinatally, to children who are at risk. The reluctance of the present British government to initiate universal HBV vaccination for newborns increases the risk of vertical transmission.

Body fluids (non-sexual transmission)

The most common setting for exchange of body fluids is almost certainly unprotected penetrative sex, probably followed by perinatal micro-transfusion; these are dealt with above, this section is concerned with other circumstances in which parenteral exposures to infected body fluids may occur.

A number of the viral infections known to be associated with cancer are found in the blood, and sometimes other body fluids, of infected individuals. There was, at one time, a significant risk of acquiring such an infection from routine transfusion of either whole blood or blood products, screening of donors and of units has reduced this risk to a negligible level; in the two decades from 1984 to 2005 the risk of HIV from transfusion fell from greater than 1 in 1 000 to less than 1 in 1 000 000[32].

Blood transfusion was a major route of spread of hepatitis B and C prior to introduction of effective screening of donated blood, in the 1990s[33]. In routine clinical practice the risk of transmission of any known viruses by transfusion is now extremely small; the risk of cancer as a consequence of transfusion-transmitted infection (TTI) is almost non-existent[34-37]. It is, by definition, impossible to exclude the possibility that there may be a yet unidentified transfusion-transmissible infectious agent. A potential defence against such agents is treatment of blood and blood products with processes which neutralize all nucleic-acid based organisms; this approach is not infallible, however, as it is ineffective against certain viruses and against intra-cellular pathogens[32].

Iatrogenic spread of viral infections continues to be a significant risk in may parts of the developing world; either from transfusions – given a lack of donor screening and payment of donors, or from repeated use of single-use equipment or inadequate sterilization of reusable equipment. Egypt has one of the world's highest hepatitis C rates; a consequence of transmission of hepatitis C during the parenteral anti-schistosomiasis therapy programme, which may have led to '*the world's largest iatrogenic transmission of blood-borne pathogens*'[38]. Anyone travelling to a country where the risk of iatrogenic infection is high may be advised to purchase a kit containing sterile needles, syringes and fluid-giving sets.

There have been conflicting reports on whether transfusion increases the risk of non-Hodgkin lymphoma, or of other cancers by mechanisms other than infection transmission. An excess of tobacco- and alcohol-related cancers in blood transfusion recipients may indicate high-risk lifestyles increase the hazard ratios both for needing transfusion and developing cancer[39]. A theoretical mechanism is transfusion-related immunomodulation (TRIM); a state of relative immunosuppression induced by transfusion of leukocyte-containing blood products. Prior to the AIDS pandemic, it was routine to allotransfuse prospective renal transplant recipients to reduce the risk of graft rejection[40]. A recent review of TRIM concluded that it is not a clinically significant problem[41]. Existing evidence does not support any role of transfusion in cancer aetiology beyond the well-characterized mechanism of transfusion-transmitted viral infection.

In the early years of public awareness of HIV/AIDS there were press reports of exaggerated precautions taken in situations in which virus transmission was extremely unlikely[42]. Interestingly, laboratory personnel, who deal with blood and body fluids on a daily basis, were less prone to AIDS hysteria as they were already accustomed to taking precautions against hepatitis B virus. Even today, when HIV is much commoner in the general population, hepatitis B represents a much higher risk. Hepatitis B is more common than HIV, with 1 in 3 of the world's population having been infected at some time; it is up to 100 times more infectious than HIV; and is much hardier than HIV, surviving for up to 7 days outside the body[43]. HBV (and HCV) can, unlike HIV, be spread by sharing of utensils like toothbrushes or razors which are contaminated with infected blood. Sharing of needles and/or syringes, a common practice with i.v. drug users, can readily transmit HBV. In the domestic environment, as in the clinical, adequate precautions against HBV transmission will offer complete protection against other body-fluid borne infections, including HIV.

Spread of blood-borne viruses in prisons is exacerbated by the refusal to provide sterile needles and syringes (as for condoms, it is argued this would condone illegal behaviour) – this is out of step with the policy of many other countries. Experience in other countries pursing a more enlightened policy has shown marked decreases in needle sharing, no further cases of HIV or Hep B and no reports of needles used as weapons once needle exchange schemes are in place[44,45]. Sexual transmission *may* occur between women but in female prisons the primary mode of spread is sharing of drug paraphernalia. All males who have served custodial sentences must be regarded as high-risk, as must all female i.v. drug users who have been in prison.

Post-transplant lymphoproliferative disorder (PTLD)

A special circumstance exists following a solid organ or haematopoietic stem cell transplant; while the recipient is receiving immunosuppressive therapy to prevent graft rejection. In this situation, the recipient may develop a virus-driven lymphoproliferative disorder, a complication first described in 1969[46,47]. Almost all early post-transplant lymphoproliferative disorder (PTLD) is thought to be EBV-related as is a proportion of late PTLD – late PTLD is typically monoclonal and more probably represents a true malignancy, unlike early cases which are polyclonal expansions of latently EBV-infected memory B cells[48].

Many PTLD arise in an existing host population of EBV-infected cells, which is unsurprising, given that over 90% of adults are EBV-positive. In about 50% of cases the tumour cells in PTLD are EBV-negative – it is thought that, in the early stages almost all PTLD is driven by latent viral infections, often EBV but also including CMV[49].

In cases, usually in paediatric patients, where a recipient is EBV-negative there may be a symptomatic phase resembling infectious mononucleosis (glandular fever) – this represents the initial infection with EBV[49]. It is extremely improbable that an EBV-negative transplant candidate would be found a tissue-matched EBV-negative donor. Fortunately, evidence suggests that in this group PTLD will often resolve following reduction in the level of immunosuppression[49]; the principal risk of this approach is rejection of the transplanted organ/tissue.

Options for prevention

It is at least theoretically possible that some infections associated with cancer could be eradicated. The successful elimination of smallpox in the wild led to optimistic predictions that many other diseases would follow the same path; unfortunately these ignored the special features of smallpox which had made eradication feasible. These include:

- Smallpox is not infectious prior to appearance of visible lesions
- Post-exposure vaccination may prevent infection or, at least, reduce severity of disease and probability of onward transmission
- Diagnosis and confirmation of smallpox cases does not require sophisticated, and expensive, laboratory facilities
- Smallpox is not highly contagious – brief exposure is unlikely to lead to infection
- There is no non-human reservoir for the disease and there is no chronic carrier state
- Vaccination protects individuals for years making it feasible to interrupt transmission

These features mean that, once a high degree of herd immunity had been achieved, it was possible to establish a surveillance programme with prompt isolation of new cases and post-exposure vaccination of contacts.

Unfortunately, none of the infections causally linked to cancer have enough of these features to make eradication a realistic policy. It has been suggested that it may be feasible to eradicate *H. pylori* infection, but this is not universally accepted as a desirable goal.

Primary prevention – blocking transmission

This is feasible for parasite infestations as all those relevant to human cancer have life cycles which require infection of non-human intermediate hosts. It is theoretically possible to completely break the life cycle of the parasite, either by eradication of secondary hosts or by preventing secondary hosts from becoming infected.

Schistosome species

These are transmitted when infectious forms of the parasite are released into fresh water by the intermediate host, a water snail. The necessary conditions for spread are, therefore:

■ Contamination of the water supply by faeces or urine from a population of chronically infected individuals
■ The presence of water snails capable of acting as hosts for the relevant species of Schistosome
■ Exposure of unprotected human skin to contaminated water

Initially, attention was focused on removal of the intermediate host – the water snail – by use of molluscicides, but these are expensive, complex to use and highly toxic to other aquatic species[50]. The introduction of safe, affordable schistosomicides changed the emphasis to morbidity control through population-based chemotherapy. Affordable is a relative term, the preferred drug is praziquantel, but, in the regions where schistosomiasis is endemic, even this is deemed relatively expensive at around 5p per average dose[51]. The simplest protective measure is good sanitation preventing infection of water and education about the risks associated with bathing in infected waters; a common problem with this approach is the lack of any practicable alternative[52].

Helicobacter pylori

In light of its status as an International Agency for Research on Cancer (IARC) class I carcinogen[53], it has been proposed that 'The only good Helicobacter pylori is a dead Helicobacter pylori'[54]. An alternative view holds that since H. pylori and humans have co-evolved[55], it may be more accurate to regard H. pylori not as a pathogen, or even just a commensal, but as a symbiont[56]. In particular, Blaser points to the increased incidence of certain GI conditions, including cancers in H. pylori free populations[57]. There is an inverse relationship between incidence of conditions linked to gastric hyperacidity and H. pylori infection rates.

There is a strong consensus that patients who have symptoms attributable to H. pylori infection should receive specific antibacterial therapy to eradicate the bacterium. Many experts argue that different policies should be adopted in the developed and developing worlds for population level eradication campaigns against H. pylori. In the developing world, H. pylori infection is extremely common and gastric cancer is a leading cause of death – here the benefits of eradication appear unchallengeable. In the developed world the incidence of gastric cancer is relatively low and has been falling for many years – the benefits of eradication programmes in these populations are far more questionable.

This is especially so when one considers that the incidence of infection with H. pylori is already on the wane in developed countries. A further reason for challenging the case for eradication in this latter population is the evidence for a reduced incidence of certain upper GI cancers in patients who are infected with *H. pylori*. Furthermore, a population level campaign would require treatment of asymptomatic individuals with antibiotics – a practice which might exacerbate the problem of antibiotic resistance in pathogenic species. Many infections seen in the hospital setting are already multiply antibiotic resistant and this has been identified as a serious public health problem.

Virus infections

Although some viruses may not be entirely species-specific, they do not have complex life cycles or intermediate hosts, which would facilitate their elimination in the wild. Eradication of smallpox in the wild depended on very specific features of the disease, and is unlikely to be repeatable for any other viral infection. The primary consideration in blocking transmission of viral infection in the general population is use of health education to achieve changes in behaviour of potential hosts. For ubiquitous viruses like EBV, it is unlikely that this would be feasible for most people; vertical transmission of infections such as hepatitis B makes it difficult to limit spread in the developing world.

Many religious movements, of various denominations, have opposed HPV vaccination, arguing that, because condoms use offers incomplete protection, fidelity campaigns are just as effective. These campaigns rely on commitment by young women to remain virgin until they marry and to remain monogamous, thereafter. The evidence suggests that any degree of success for such campaigns requires that they can guarantee total abstinence by both partners before marriage and total monogamy by both partners during marriage[58]. Even this may not be sufficient, in light of evidence of non-sexual transmission of HPV during childhood[18]. A number of reviews have compared 'abstinence only' policies – in which no advice is given on safe-sex, condom use, etc. – and 'abstinence plus' sometimes referred to as ABC;

- Abstinence from sexual intercourse before marriage
- Being faithful within marriage
- Condom use

Reviews have tended to demonstrate greater efficacy for abstinence plus or objective sex education without abstinence advocacy as compared with abstinence only; the president of the US Institute of Medicine testified before a Congressional committee to the effect that *'abstinence-only programs do not reduce the risk of HIV as measured by self-reported behavioral outcomes......Comprehensive sex-education programs appear more promising. Several studies found a positive effect on a number of behavioral outcomes'*[59]. Although the studies were addressing behaviour influencing HIV risk, this may be taken as a surrogate for reduction in risk of other sexually-transmitted conditions.

The history of campaigns against STIs suggests that prevention based on health education will have, at best, a very limited role in primary prevention. The assumption must be made for most viral infections that exposure will continue at the same levels as historically. Prevention will depend on blocking infection following exposure.

Attempts to prevent vertical transmission of virus infections, in the course of breast-feeding, have been more successful. The most striking success has been in Japan, where this route of infection has been virtually eliminated for HTLV-1[6]; this achievement was possible because in developed countries, such as Japan, it is safe to substitute bottle-feeding in place of breast-feeding. In the developing world, lack of safe water supplies has meant that bottle-feeding has been associated with high risk of death due to infectious disease.

Mother-to-child transmission of HIV is an important problem in developing countries. Extensive programmes have been established for prevention of mother-to-child transmission (PMTCT); the most successful element of this has been treatment of HIV-positive women with antiretroviral drugs, starting from the 18th week of pregnancy, which addresses both intrauterine infection and perinatal infection. In the developing world mortality from formula feed-associated infection is greater than from HIV, especially if neonatal antiretroviral therapy is given; it has been clearly shown that, in these circumstances, the safest option is exclusive breast-feeding for at least 6 months[60,61]. Mixed breast-feeding (combining breast feeding with formula or with solids before 6 months) was associated with a higher level of HIV infection – possible causes include alterations in the gut defences and presence of protective fatty acids in breast milk which are inactivated by mixed feeding.

Primary prevention – enhancing host resistance

The most common and most significant infectious causes of cancer, certainly in the developed world, are viral infections. Since it is unlikely that major progress can be made in blocking exposure of the population to viral agents, prevention will depend on measures to enhance host resistance. There has been considerable success in several populations in reducing prevalence of virus infections by immunization. A major topic of debate is the extent to which programmes should differ between developing countries in which such infections are commonly endemic and often vertically transmitted, and the developed world where the individual risk of infection is much lower. Population level data in developed countries may be misleading, with low overall levels concealing the existence of subgroups with prevalence more typical of developing world population. In this context there may be a case for programmes of selective immunization to target at-risk populations.

Hepatitis viruses

In a prescient editorial in the *BMJ*[62], it was predicted that, '*While the control of acute infectious hepatitis by vaccination remains unattainable the disease will probably continue to cause large epidemics throughout the world'*. The *BMJ* comment predated the identification of HBV as the causal agent of infectious hepatitis[63], and the development of an effective safe vaccine. Probably the most extensive global vaccination programme to date has been of that against hepatitis B. A programme of infant immunization in Taiwan reduced the incidence fourfold[64] from 0.52 to 0.13 per 100 000. A global campaign, endorsed by WHO, has seen immunization cover expand from 15% in 1996 to 60% in 2006[65]. This is likely to be of critical importance to reducing the incidence of hepatocellular carcinoma (HCC) in endemic areas, as early infection confers a much higher risk of cirrhosis compared with adult-acquired infection. A recent paper summarizes the updated (2010) WHO recommendations on use of hepatitis B vaccines[66]. The UK failed to follow the WHO recommendation, adopting a policy of selective vaccination of high-risk populations and of infants born to high-risk mothers, a 2004 *BMJ* review stated, *'The United Kingdom is one of the few developed countries that have not implemented universal neonatal hepatitis B immunisation. ….It is time that this policy is reviewed in the light of experience with selective immunisation, data on efficacy of universal immunisation from other countries, and the proved safety of recombinant vaccines'*[67]. In 2007 the BMA voted to ask the DoH to *'introduce the hepatitis B vaccine into the childhood schedule without further delay'*[68].

A major opportunity to limit spread of adult blood-borne viruses (BBV) in the UK is being rejected on political grounds. The measures needed to reduce spread of BBV in the prison population are known and have been shown to work in jurisdictions where they have been introduced, yet the Prison Service refuses to countenance their application in UK prisons. They are free confidential provision of condoms to protect against sexual transmission and provision of needle exchange schemes to avoid transmission by sharing of drug paraphernalia. These measures are rejected in the UK on the grounds that prisoners are breaking the law in engaging in sexual activity or taking drugs and provision of condoms or safe injecting paraphernalia would condone such criminal acts. The prison medical service are mandated to provide condoms to prisoners at risk of HIV infection, while disinfecting tablets are available to reduce risks of sharing injection equipment; unfortunately, in both cases to request access to these services is to admit to breaking prison rules and risks stigmatization of the inmate.

Given the unfortunate stance of the Prison Service in blocking the most effective harm reduction options, it is fortunate that most, but not all, prisoners are offered HBV vaccination. This is of particular importance given the documented high risk of sexual assault in prison. A recent study[69] stated that 2% of a sample of 208 prisoner participants had had forced penetrative sexual intercourse; this would indicate almost 2000 victims in the UK prison system at any given time. Many prisoners are i.v. drug users prior to admission but, while they may have used risk-reduction prior to incarceration, this is not possible in prison. An unfortunate reported result of mandatory drug testing has been a switch by prisoners from cannabis (which persists in the body) to heroin use, which can only be detected for a short period after intake[70].

Unfortunately, there is presently no vaccine available against hepatitis C; prevention is restricted to measures to minimize exposure to the virus – these are the same as are indicated for hepatitis B or HIV. The total dependence of hepatitis D on HBV for replication and transmission means that effective control of HBV offers HDV eradication as a bonus – 'buy one get one free'.

Papillomaviruses

There are many papillomavirus species which infect humans (HPV), but fortunately most of these are not considered high-risk for cancer. The most prevalent HPV-associated cancer is cancer of the cervix; this is one of the commonest cancers in the developed world and, in much of the developing world, is the leading cause of cancer death. Two high-risk strains, HPV 16 and 18 are considered to account for around 70% of cases of cervical cancer, which kills about 250 000 women each year, globally[71]. Infection occurs in a very high proportion of sexually active women, but in most cases a highly effective local immune response eliminates the virus within 2 years[72]. Although condom use appears to reduce the risk of HPV infection, this protection is not complete – the reduction in risk has been estimated to be around 70%[19].

A major reduction in cervical cancer mortality in the developed world was achieved by screening programmes to detect and treat pre-malignant stages of the disease. The basis for such screening has been exfoliative cytology, first developed in 1928 by Papanicolaou[73], and in widespread use by the 1960s in many developed countries. Prior to the introduction of the smear or 'Pap test', rates of death from cervical cancer in developed countries matched those now only seen in the developing world[74,75]. Although the screening programme has offered great benefits, it is difficult to implement in the developing world as it requires laboratory facilities and skilled staff, which are rarely available; to prevent invasive cancer, surgical treatment of early lesions is necessary and this too is often infeasible in developing countries[76].

There have been developments of screening, using techniques such as HPV DNA detection, but these are still probably beyond the reaches of countries where cervical cancer mortality is greatest. A major development in this area is the introduction of vaccines designed to protect against the highest-risk types of HPV[77]– these have now been introduced into clinical practice in the developed world[78], but not without a great deal of controversy[79]. Among the important issues raised are:

- Choice of vaccine – divalent versus quadrivalent
- Timing of vaccination – seen by some as legitimizing early sexualization
- Target population – girls only or boys as well (oral cancer, anal cancer, genital polyps)
- Efficacy and safety – allegations that the effectiveness and safety of the virus have been 'over-hyped'

■ Compulsion – should vaccination be mandated or voluntary
■ Should the vaccine be offered to older women – efficacy in sexually active women
■ Screening policy – how, if at all, should screening policies be modified

In the US, and many other countries, the vaccine licensed for general use in young females is Gardasil™, which protects against four strains, HPV 16 and 18, which are thought to account for about 70% of cervical cancer, and also HPV 6 and 11, which cause 90% of anogenital warts[80].

Most scientists and health-care workers believe it preferable to vaccinate early, before women become sexually active; against this are ranged some who are against vaccination at any age, believing it would promote promiscuity, and others who are against early vaccination, for fear this would invite premature sexual activity.

An ideal vaccination strategy would probably include boys because this would reduce the chance of them becoming carriers and eventually passing on the infection to female partners. Inclusion of HPV 6/11 was expected to improve willingness of parents of boys to give consent for use of a vaccine which would protect the recipient; as boys are at low risk of HPV 16/18-related disease they would derive less benefit from a vaccine containing only those strains.

In the UK the Department of Health, against the advice of most experts, chose the cheaper divalent vaccine Cervarix™, which protects only against the HPV 16 and 18 strains. Although anogenital warts do not carry the high mortality of cervical cancer, they can be very distressing and are considered a significant risk factor for anogenital cancer. This decision is also likely to reduce uptake if it decided in the future to extend vaccination to boys.

It has been questioned whether the evidence based on efficacy[81] and safety[82] is sufficient to justify policies of universal vaccination – especially when these are enforced by sanctions, as is the case in several US states[83]. These reports have been based on experience with Gardasil; it remains to be seen whether similar reports will emerge in relation to Cervarix.

Other viruses

Human immunodeficiency virus

After 25 years of intensive research, the Holy Grail of an effective HIV vaccine remains as elusive as ever. It has been pointed out that it took as long to develop an effective vaccine against typhoid and almost twice as long to create vaccines against measles and polio[84]. For the foreseeable future, blocking transmission will continue to be the most important component of HIV/AIDS control.

Considerable success has been achieved by schemes to persuade men who have sex with men (MSM) to substitute safer sex in place of high-risk behaviour.

Epstein–Barr virus

Epstein-Barr virus (EBV), is possibly the most ubiquitous infectious organism in the human population – levels of current or past infection are consistently estimated to be well in excess of 90%. In the overwhelming majority of cases, EBV infection causes either no illness at all or a mild flu-like pyrexial condition. In a minority of cases in the Western world, when acquired in teenage or young-adult life, it may cause a condition called glandular fever – this is still benign in almost all cases. In the developing world Epstein–Barr virus is believed to be a major causal factor for Burkitt lymphoma. There are several other forms of cancer for which EBV is believed to be a significant risk factor. zur Hausen has estimated the EBV-linked global cancer burden as over 200 000 cases per year[85].

In light of the range of associated cancers, and the estimated disease burden, there have been proposals for a vaccination campaign to eliminate EBV. This might be attractive in terms of benefit to the developed world but it is extraordinarily ambitious, both in light of the biology of EBV and of the variability in clinical consequences of the infection. As previously cited, there are a number of features of smallpox which account for the relative ease with which it was eradicated; almost all of the relevant features of EBV are the precise opposite, probably rendering eradication infeasible. Smallpox was a significant cause of death and serious illness in the developed world at the start of the campaign for eradication, being highly infectious and having a high mortality. EBV-related cancers, in contrast, are very uncommon in the developed world and cause few deaths in the general population. A successful vaccination campaign would require a global vaccination programme and, in the developed world, this would probably cause more morbidity than EBV. Given the relative indifference of Western populations to famine in developing nations, it seems unlikely that altruism would lead to a significant uptake. It is possible, if a safe, effective vaccine is developed, that local campaigns in the developing world might impact on the burden of Burkitt's lymphoma. Even here, it is probable that a better investment of resources might be a vaccine against malarial infection.

Given that EBV-associated malignancies usually (always?) arise against a background of immunosuppression, it may well be that the most effective form of prevention would be to address the underlying mechanisms for immunoparesis.

KSHV/HHV-8

The principal mechanism of transmission of HHV-8 has not been clearly determined. It is present most commonly and at highest levels in saliva[86], suggesting that non-sexual intimate contact may be sufficient for infection to occur. Although it has been shown in an African study to be transmissible by transfusion[87], special features present in this study population suggest that the risk from transfusion in non-endemic areas is very low; although prevention of transfusional transmission is theoretically possible, this may not be feasible in the endemic areas.

References

1. O'Toole, L., Nurse, P. & Radda, G. (2003) An analysis of cancer research funding in the UK. *Nature Reviews. Cancer*, **3**, 139–143.

2. Laurance, J. (22 October 2002) Analysis: Map reveals the cancers which the public do not care about. *Independent,* London.

3. Department of Health (2007) *Cancer Reform Strategy*. Department of Health, London.

4. Parker, H.W., Varma, R.R., Rothwell, D.J. & Borkowf, H.I. (1976) Venereal transmission of hepatitis B virus. The possible role of vaginal secretions. *Obstetrics & Gynecology*, **48**, 410–412.

5. Kourtis, A.P., Lee, F.K., Abrams, E.J., Jamieson, D.J. & Bulterys, M. (2006) Mother-to-child transmission of HIV-1: Timing and implications for prevention. *The Lancet Infectious Diseases*, **6**, 726–732.

6. Kashiwagi, K., Furusyo, N., Nakashima, H., Kubo, N., Kinukawa, N., Kashiwagi, S. & Hayashi, J. (2004) A decrease in mother-to-child transmission of human T lymphotropic virus type I (HTLV-I) in Okinawa, Japan. *The American Journal of Tropical Medicine and Hygiene*, **70**, 158–163.

7. Garg, P.K., Perry, S., Sanchez, L. & Parsonnet, J. (2006) Concordance of *Helicobacter pylori* infection among children in extended-family homes. *Epidemiology and Infection*, **134**, 450–459.

8. Foundation for Liver Research (October 2004) *Hepatitis B: Out of the Shadows: A Report into the Impact of Hepatitis B on the Nation's Health*. Foundation for Liver Research, London.

9. Pungpapong, S., Kim, W.R. & Poterucha, J.J. (2007) Natural history of hepatitis B virus infection: An update for clinicians. *Mayo Clinic Proceedings*, **82**, 967–975.

10. Straus, S.E., Cohen, J.I., Tosato, G. & Meier, J. (1993) NIH conference. Epstein–Barr virus infections: Biology, pathogenesis, and management. *Annals of Internal Medicine*, **118**, 45–58.

11. Bornkamm, G.W., Behrends, U. & Mautner, J. (2006) The infectious kiss: Newly infected B cells deliver Epstein–Barr virus to epithelial cells. *PNAS*, **103**, 7201–7202.

12. Williams, H. & Crawford, D.H. (2006) Epstein–Barr virus: The impact of scientific advances on clinical practice. *Blood*, **107**, 862–869.

13. Marrazzo, J.M., Coffey, P. & Bingham, A. (2005) Sexual practices, risk perception and knowledge of sexually transmitted disease risk among lesbian and bisexual women. *Perspectives on Sexual and Reproductive Health*, **37**, 6–12.

14. Marrazzo, J.M. (2004) Barriers to infectious disease care among lesbians. *Emerging Infectious Diseases*, **10**, 1974–1978.

15. Szajerka, T. & Jablecki, J. (2007) Kaposi's sarcoma revisited. *AIDS Reviews*, **9**, 3–10.

16. Dodds, J. & Mercey, D. (2006) *Sexual Health Survey of Gay Men in London 2005: Annual Summary Report*. Centre for Sexual Health and HIV Research, University College London, London.

17. Elford, J., Bolding, G., Sherr, L. & Hart, G. (2005) High-risk sexual behaviour among London gay men: No longer increasing. *AIDS*, **19**, 2171–2174.

18. Sinclair, K.A., Woods, C.R., Kirse, D.J. & Sinal, S.H. (2005) Anogenital and respiratory tract human papillomavirus infections among children: Age, gender, and potential transmission through sexual abuse. *Pediatrics*, **116**, 815–825.

19. Winer, R.L., Hughes, J.P., Feng, Q., O'Reilly, S., Kiviat, N.B., Holmes, K.K. & Koutsky, L.A. (2006) Condom use and the risk of genital human papillomavirus infection in young women. *The New England Journal of Medicine*, **354**, 2645–2654.

20. Hernandez, B.Y., Wilkens, L.R., Zhu, X., Thompson, P., McDuffie, K., Shvetsov, Y.B., Kamemoto, L.E., Killeen, J., Ning, L. & Goodman, M.T. (2008) Transmission of human papillomavirus in heterosexual couples. *Emerging Infectious Diseases*, **14**, 888–894.

21. Ault, K.A. (2006) Epidemiology and natural history of human papillomavirus infections in the female genital tract. *Infectious Diseases in Obstetrics and Gynecology*, **2006**, 40475. doi: 10.1155/IDOG/2006/40470.

22. Bosch, F.X. & de Sanjose, S. (2007) The epidemiology of human papillomavirus infection and cervical cancer. *Disease Markers*, **23**, 213–227.

23. Starnbach, M.N. & Roan, N.R. (2008) Conquering sexually transmitted diseases. *Nature Reviews. Immunology*, **8**, 313–317.

24. Szmuness, W. (1975) Recent advances in the study of the epidemiology of hepatitis B. *The American Journal of Pathology*, **81**, 629–650.

25. Mast, E.E., Weinbaum, C.M., Fiore, A.E., Alter, M.J., Bell, B.P., Finelli, L., Rodewald, L.E., Douglas, J.M. Jr., Janssen, R.S. & Ward, J.W. (2006) A comprehensive immunization strategy to eliminate transmission of hepatitis B virus infection in the United States: Recommendations of the Advisory Committee on Immunization Practices (ACIP) Part II: Immunization of adults. *MMWR Recommendations and Reports*, **55**, 1–33.

26. Cavalheiro, N.P. (2007) Sexual transmission of hepatitis C. *Revista do Instituto de Medicina Tropical de São Paulo*, **49**, 271–277.

27. Zignego, A.L., Fontana, R., Puliti, S., Barbagli, S., Monti, M., Careccia, G., Giannelli, F., Buzzelli, G., Brunetto, M.R. et al. (1997) Relevance of inapparent coinfection by hepatitis B virus in alpha interferon-treated patients with hepatitis C virus chronic hepatitis. *Journal of Medical Virology*, **51**, 313–318.

28. Hsieh, T.H., Liu, C.J., Chen, D.S. & Chen, P.J. (2006) Natural course and treatment of hepatitis D virus infection. *Journal of the Formosan Medical Association*, **105**, 869–881.

29. Kao, J.H. & Chen, D.S. (2002) Recent updates in hepatitis vaccination and the prevention of hepatocellular carcinoma. *International Journal of Cancer*, **97**, 269–271.

30. Edgar, K., Azad, Y. & Valette, D. (2005) *HIV and Hepatitis in UK Prisons: Addressing Prisoners' Healthcare Needs*. Prison Reform Trust/National AIDS Trust, London.

31. Palmer, I. (2003) Sexuality and soldiery: Combat & condoms, continence & cornflakes. *Journal of the Royal Army Medical Corps*, **149**, 38–46.

32. Blajchman, M.A. & Vamvakas, E.C. (2006) The continuing risk of transfusion-transmitted infections. *The New England Journal of Medicine*, **355**, 1303–1305.

33. Centers for Disease Control and Prevention (1998) Recommendations for prevention and control of hepatitis C virus (HCV) infection and HCV-related chronic disease. *MMWR Recommendations and Reports*, **47**, 1–39.

34. Otsubo, H. & Yamaguchi, K. (2008) Current risks in blood transfusion in Japan. *Japanese Journal of Infectious Diseases*, **61**, 427–433.

35. Canadian Paediatric Society. (2006) Transfusion and risk of infection in Canada: Update 2006. *The Canadian Journal of Infectious Diseases & Medical Microbiology*, **17**, 103–107.

36. Madjdpour, C., Heindl, V. & Spahn, D.R. (2006) Risks, benefits, alternatives and indications of allogenic blood transfusions. *Minerva Anestesiol*, **72**, 283–298.

37. Kaur, P. & Basu, S. (2005) Transfusion-transmitted infections: Existing and emerging pathogens. *Journal of Postgraduate Medicine*, **51**, 146–151.

38. Frank, C., Mohamed, M.K., Strickland, G.T., Lavanchy, D., Arthur, R.R., Magder, L.S. et al. (2000) The role of parenteral antischistosomal therapy in the spread of hepatitis C virus in Egypt. *Lancet*, **355**, 887–891.

39. Hjalgrim, H., Edgren, G., Rostgaard, K., Reilly, M., Tran, T.N., Titlestad, K.E., Shanwell, A., Jersild, C., Adami, J., Wikman, A., Gridley, G., Wideroff, L., Nyren, O. & Melbye, M. (2007) Cancer incidence in blood transfusion recipients. *Journal of the National Cancer Institute*, **99**, 1864–1874.

40. Opelz, G., Sengar, D.P., Mickey, M. R. et al. (1973) Effect of blood transfusion on subsequent kidney transplants. *Transplantation Proceedings*, **5**, 253–259.

41. Vamvakas, E.C. & Blajchman, M.A. (2007) Transfusion-related immunomodulation (TRIM): An update. *Blood Reviews*, **21**, 327–348.

42. Times reporter. (9 November 1985) Aids scare in court. *The Times*, London.

43. So, S. (2007) *2007 Physician's Guide to HBV: A Silent Killer*. Asian Liver Center, San Francisco, CA.

44. Okie, S. (2007) Sex, drugs, prisons, and HIV. *The New England Journal of Medicine*, **356**, 105–108.

45. Dolan, K., Rutter, S. & Wodak, A.D. (2003) Prison-based syringe exchange programmes: A review of international research and development. *Addiction*, **98**, 153–158.

46. Penn, I., Hammond, W. & Brettschneidter, L. (1969) Malignant lymphomas in transplantation patients. *Transplantation Proceedings*, **1**, 106–112.

47. McKhann, C.F. (1969) Primary malignancy in patients undergoing immunosuppression for renal transplantation. *Transplantation*, **8**, 209–212.

48. Carbone, A, Gloghini, A. & Dotti, G. (2008) EBV-associated lymphoproliferative disorders: Classification and treatment. *Oncologist*, **13**, 577–585.

49. Trappe, R., Oertel, S. & Riess, H. (2006) Pathogenetic, clinical, diagnostic and therapeutic aspects of post-transplantation lymphoproliferative disorders. *Deutsches Ärzteblatt*, **103**, 3259–3267.

50. Gryseels, B., Polman, K., Clerinx, J. & Kestens, L. (2006) Human schistosomiasis. *Lancet*, **368**, 1106–1118.

51. Crompton, D.W.T & WHO (2006) *Preventive Chemotherapy in Human Helminthiasis: Coordinated Use of Antihelminthic Drugs in Control Interventions: A Manual for Health Professionals and Programme Managers*. World Health Organization, Geneva.

52. Ekeh, H.E. & Adeniyi, J.D. (1998) Health education strategies for tropical disease control in school children, *The Journal of Tropical Medicine and Hygiene*, **91**, 55–59.

53. IARC. (1994) Schistosomes, liver flukes and *Helicobacter pylori*. IARC Working Group on the Evaluation of Carcinogenic Risks to Humans. Lyon, 7–14 June 1994. *IARC Monographs on the Evaluation of Carcinogenic Risks to Humans*, **61**, 1–241.

54. Graham, D.Y. (1997) The only good *Helicobacter pylori* is a dead *Helicobacter pylori*. *Lancet* **350**, 70–71.

55. Linz, B., Balloux, F., Moodley, Y., Manica, A., Liu, H., Roumagnac, P., Falush, D., Stamer, C., Prugnolle, F., van der Merwe, S.W., Yamaoka, Y., Graham, D.Y., Perez-Trallero, E., Wadstrom, T., Suerbaum, S. & Achtman, M. (2007) An African origin for the intimate association between humans and *Helicobacter pylori*. *Nature*, **445**, 915–918.

56. Blaser, M.J. (2006) Who are we? Indigenous microbes and the ecology of human diseases. *EMBO Reports*, **7**, 956–960.

57. Blaser, M.J. (1999) Hypothesis: The changing relationships of *Helicobacter pylori* and humans: Implications for health and disease. *The Journal of Infectious Diseases*, **179**, 1523–1530.

58. Weaver, B.A. (2006) Epidemiology and natural history of genital human papillomavirus infection. *The Journal of the American Osteopathic Association*, **106**, S2–S8.

59. Fineberg, H.V. (2008) *Statement on Effectiveness of Sex Education Programs before the Committee on Oversight and Government Reform of the U.S. House of Representatives*. U.S. Government, Washington, DC.

60. Coovadia, H.M., Rollins, N., Bland, R.M., Little, K., Coutsoudis, A., Bennish, M.L. & Newell, M.-L. (2007) Mother-to-child transmission of HIV-1 infection during exclusive breastfeeding in the first 6 months of life: An intervention cohort study. *Lancet*, **369**, 1107–1116.

61. Kuhn, L., Sinkala, M., Kandasa, C., Semrau, K., Kasonde, P., Scott, N., Mwiya, M., Vwalika, C., Walter, J., Tsai, W-Y, Aldrovandi, G. & Thea, D.M. (2007) High uptake of exclusive breastfeeding and reduced early post-natal HIV transmission. *PLoS ONE*, **2**(12), e1363.

62. Editorial – *BMJ*. (1963) Infectious hepatitis. *BMJ*, **2**, 1602–1603.

63. Beasley, R.P. (1988) Hepatitis B virus: The major etiology of hepatocellular carcinoma. *Cancer*, **6**, 1942–1956.

64. Ni, Y.H., Huang, L.M., Chang, M.H., Yen, C.J., Lu, C.Y., You, S.L., Kao, J.H., Lin, Y.C., Chen, H.L., Hsu, H.Y. & Chen, D.S. (2007) Two decades of universal hepatitis B vaccination in Taiwan: Impact and implication for future strategies. *Gastroenterology*, **132**, 1287–1293.

65. de Martel, C. & Franceschi, S. (2009) Infections and cancer; established associations and new hypotheses. *Critical Reviews in Oncology/Hematology*, **70**, 183–194.

66. WHO Strategic Advisory Group of Experts on Immunization. (2010) Hepatitis B vaccines: WHO position paper—recommendations. *Vaccine*, **28**, 589–590.

67. Aggarwal, R. & Ranjan, P. (2004) Preventing and treating hepatitis B infection. *BMJ*, **329**, 1080–1086.

68. Pollard, A.J. (2007) Hepatitis B vaccination. *BMJ*, **335**, 950.

69. Banbury, S. (2004) Coercive sexual behaviour in British prisons as repoted by adult ex-prisoners. *The Howard Journal of Criminal Justice*, **43**, 113–130.

70. Djemil, H. (2008) *Inside Out: How to Get Drugs out of Prisons.* Centre for Policy Studies, London.

71. McIntyre, P. (2007) HPV vaccine promises much but screening remains vital. *Cancer World*, July/August, European School of Oncology, Milan, Italy, (19), 26–30.

72. Plummer, M., Schiffman, M., Castle, P.E., Maucort-Boulch, D. & Wheeler, C.M. (2007) A 2-year prospective study of human papillomavirus persistence among women with a cytological diagnosis of atypical squamous cells of undetermined significance or low-grade squamous intraepithelial lesion. *The Journal of Infectious Diseases*, **195**, 1582–1589.

73. Papanicolaou, G.N. (1928) New cancer diagnosis. *Proceedings of the Third Race Betterment Conference*, Race Betterment Foundation, Battle Creek, MI, pp. 528–534.

74. Gustafsson, L., Ponten, J., Bergstrom, R. & Adami, H.O. (1997) International incidence rates of invasive cervical cancer before cytological screening. *International Journal of Cancer*, **71**, 159–165.

75. Gustafsson, L., Ponten, J., Zack, M. & Adami, H.O. (1997) International incidence rates of invasive cervical cancer after introduction of cytological screening. *Cancer Causes & Control*, **8**, 755–763.

76. IARC Working Group on the Evaluation of Cancer Prevention Strategies (2004) Cervix cancer screening.

77. Harper, D.M., Franco, E.L., Wheeler, C., Ferris, D.G., Jenkins, D., Schuind, A., Zahaf, T., Innis, B., Naud, P., De Carvalho, N.S., Roteli-Martins, C.M., Teixeira, J., Blatter, M.M., Korn, A.P., Quint, W. & Dubin, G. (2004) Efficacy of a bivalent L1 virus-like particle vaccine in prevention of infection with human papillomavirus types 16 and 18 in young women: A randomised controlled trial. *Lancet*, **364**, 1757–1765.

78. McLemore, M.R. (2006) Gardasil: Introducing the new human papillomavirus vaccine. *Clinical Journal of Oncology Nursing*, **10**, 559–560.

79. Herzog, T.J., Huh, W.K., Downs, L.S., Smith, J.S. & Monk, B.J. (2008) Initial lessons learned in HPV vaccination. *Gynecologic Oncology*, **109**, S4–S11.

80. Gissmann, L. & zur Hausen, H. (1980) Partial characterization of viral DNA from human genital warts (condylomata acuminata). *International Journal of Cancer*, **25**, 605–609.

81. Maugh II, T.H. & Chong, J-R. (5 October 2007) Research questions worth of vaccine. *Los Angeles Times*.

82. Sikora, K. & Bissett, K. (3 December 2007) Hundreds get sick from Gardasil cancer vaccine. *Australian Daily Telegraph*.

83. Colgrove, J. (2006) The ethics and politics of compulsory HPV vaccination. *The New England Journal of Medicine*, **355**, 2389–2391.

84. Tonks, A. (2007) Quest for the AIDS vaccine. *BMJ*, **334**, 1346–1348.

85. zur Hausen, H. (2006) Infections Causing Human Cancer. Wiley-VCH, Weinheim.

86. Plancoulaine, S., Abel, L., van Beveren, M., Tregouet, D.A., Joubert, M., Tortevoye, P., de The, G. & Gessain, A. (2000) Human herpesvirus 8 transmission from mother to child and between siblings in an endemic population. *Lancet*, **356**, 1062–1065.

87. Hladik, W., Dollard, S.C., Mermin, J., Fowlkes, A.L., Downing, R., Amin, M.M., Banage, F., Nzaro, E., Kataaha, P., Dondero, T.J., Pellett, P.E. & Lackritz, E.M. (2006) Transmission of human herpesvirus 8 by blood transfusion. *The New England Journal of Medicine*, **355**, 1331–1338.

Part I   Viral Causes of Cancer

6 Herpesviruses (Herpesviridae)

Herpesviruses have closely co-evolved with vertebrates, achieving a coexistence so well adjusted that they are now described as *'ubiquitous in both human and animal populations'*[1]. Over 90% of the human population show serological evidence of current or past infection with Epstein–Barr virus. They establish lifelong latency and may reactivate after very long dormancy. Of the more than 100 known types, eight are specific to humans and thus known as human herpesviruses (HHV) – of these eight only one type (HHV-7) has no known disease association. Epstein–Barr virus (EBV) (HHV-4) and HHV-8 are classified by International Agency for Research on Cancer (IARC) as definite human carcinogens. HHV-2 (HSV-2) is a cofactor with HPV in cervical cancer[2].

With the possible exception of HHV-7, all HHV have been regarded as pathogens, or at best parasites; this relationship that has recently been reconsidered as latent herpesvirus infection has been shown (in an animal model) to upregulate the innate immune response, offering protection against bacterial infection[3].

The first confirmed viral aetiology of a human malignancy was the association between EBV infection and African endemic Burkitt's lymphoma (BL). In sub-Saharan Africa BL is the commonest childhood cancer in many areas. Although childhood BL is rare in the developed world, EBV-associated BL is a significant problem in immunosuppressed populations; this includes post-transplant lymphoproliferative disorder (PTLD).

A proportion of cases of Hodgkin lymphoma (HL) has been shown to result from EBV infection. Epidemiological evidence suggests that other HL cases may also have a viral trigger and it was believed that this could be a herpesvirus; exhaustive studies are considered to have excluded a novel herpesvirus as cause of these cases, although it is still thought likely that an infectious agent is implicated[4].

The rarity of HHV-related malignancy, set against the ubiquity of HHV infection, suggests that oncogenesis can only occur in a subset of hosts rendered vulnerable by immunosuppression. An alternative explanation, which may apply to EBV-related HL, is that timing of exposure is critical; polio infection in early childhood is trivial or subclinical but yields lifelong immunity, whereas delayed infection caused devastating neurological illness prior to widespread vaccination.

Infectious Causes of Cancer, first edition. By Ken Campbell. Published 2011 by John Wiley & Sons Ltd.
© 2011 John Wiley & Sons Ltd.

HHV-8 is geographically isolated in its distribution, rarely being seen in Europe outwith the Mediterranean regions. It is deemed a necessary, but not sufficient, cause for Kaposi sarcoma (KS) and for primary effusion lymphoma (PEL). KS is the most common AIDS-associated malignancy, whereas PEL is a very rare form of non-Hodgkin's lymphoma.

Epstein–Barr virus

The organism[5]

A gammaherpesvirus, with a 172Kb double-stranded DNA genome, which encodes for more than 100 genes, the virus persists in latently infected cells as a circular episome[6].

EBV is orally transmitted and establishes an initial lytic infection in epithelial cells and a predominantly latent infection in B-cells. Latent infection of B memory cells maintains lifelong infection. Differing patterns of gene expression are seen in lytic and latent infections and differing types of latency are associated with different malignant transformation[7].

Over 90% of the human population shows evidence of EBV transmission. Many primary infections are asymptomatic, although there may be a mild flu-like illness. Delayed primary infection may lead to glandular fever (infectious mononucleosis), sometimes referred to as 'kissing disease', reflecting the fact that in the developed world infection is often acquired from one's first boy/girlfriend. Serious illness, including malignancy, due to EBV infection is rare in the developed world; in sub-Saharan Africa EBV-related Burkitt lymphoma is the commonest malignancy in children. Nasopharyngeal carcinoma (NPC) is very variable in its geographic distribution, reflecting local exposure to cofactors.

IARC status

Group 1 – definite carcinogen in humans[8].

Associated malignancies[9,10]

The estimated annual incidence of EBV-associated cancer is around 99 000 cases of lymphoma or nasopharyngeal cancer[11], while it has been stated that EBV is found in about 10% of gastric adenocarcinomas, which amounts to around 75 000 cases per year[5]. Table 6.1 lists cancers classed by IARC as EBV-related[12] and those others which have been reported to contain EBV and in each case indicates the percentage reported to contain EBV virus[9].

The most important of these, in the developed world, are Hodgkin's lymphoma, non-Hodgkin's lymphoma, Burkitt's lymphoma in immunosuppressed patients and post-transplant lymphoproliferative disorder.

Table 6.1 Proportion of various cancers reported to be EBV positive.

Malignancy	Subtype	EBV-positive (%)
Burkitt's lymphoma	Endemic	>95
	Non-endemic	15–30
Hodgkin lymphoma	Mixed cellularity	70
	Lymphocyte depleted	>95
	Nodular sclerosing	10–40
	Lymphocyte predominant	<5
Non-Hodgkin lymphoma	Nasal T/NK	>90
	Angioimmunoblastic lymphadenopathy	Unknown
Post-transplant lymphoproliferative disorder		>90
AIDS-associated lymphoma	IP-CNS	>95
Nasopharyngeal carcinoma	Anaplastic	>95

The following malignancies are not listed by IARC as caused by EBV, but have been reported to be EBV-positive in at least some cases

Malignancy	Subtype	EBV-positive (%)
Breast cancer	Medullary carcinoma Adenocarcinoma	0–50
Gastric cancer	Lymphoepithelioma-like	>90
	Adenocarcinoma	5–25
	Other	30–50
Leiomyosarcoma in immunosuppressed patients		Frequent

Hodgkin's lymphoma[13–16]

Hodgkin's lymphoma (HL) is defined by the presence of the distinctive Reed–Sternberg cell. It is highly atypical among cancers in that the malignant cell population is heavily outnumbered by an inflammatory infiltrate; this is so striking that for many years it was disputed whether it was a reactive condition or a true malignancy[17]. It is thought probable that HL represents a disease complex, rather than a single condition; there are probably three different types of EBV-associated HL and another non-EBV-related group[18]. It is possible to demonstrate EBV in HL cells in about 40% of cases[19]. Several extensive reviews have been published of the biology of HL and of its relationship with EBV[15,18,20–24].

Burkitt's lymphoma[25–29]

Burkitt's lymphoma (BL), the discovery of which has been described in detail in Chapter 1, is rare in immunocompetent persons. Almost all endemic cases are EBV positive[26], although they are thought to have a complex aetiology involving multiple cofactors[27,30,31]. In developed countries, it is seen most frequently in HIV positive and other immunocompromised populations. The clinical presentation of these cases is distinct from that of endemic or 'African' BL; endemic BL typically presents with jaw tumour, often bilateral at diagnosis, while non-endemic cases often present as abdominal lymphoma[21,32,33].

BL is typically highly chemosensitive, and effective short duration, high-intensity multi-drug regimens have been devised which are well suited to use in countries with low-level health-care resources[29].

Post-transplant lymphoproliferative disorder[10,34–36]

Post-transplant lymphoproliferative disorder (PTLD) occurs as a consequence of iatrogenic immunosuppression following therapeutic transplantation. The nature of the risk and the management of the condition are highly dependent on the nature of the transplant and on the immunosuppression. There is an extensive literature on PTLD in different contexts[10,35,37–46].

Cofactors

EBV-associated cancer typically occurs in immunosuppressed individuals. The most plausible mechanism is disruption of normal mechanisms restricting the B-cell response to antigenic stimulation, which allows immortalized EBV-positive B-cells to proliferate. The ubiquity of EBV in human populations means that a high proportion of immunodeficiency-associated cancers are EBV positive. The great majority of post-transplant lymphoproliferative disorders are EBV positive; in some of these cases (particularly in children), control can be gained by reduction of iatrogenic immunosuppression, although this risks loss of the transplanted organ(s); in adult patients, chemotherapy may be effective but is more toxic than in patients with a primary diagnosis of LPD[46].

Extensive research is focused on developing specific immunotherapies targeting EBV-positive cells; this approach might be effective against all associated malignancies[47]. Current studies use EBV-specific cytotoxic T lymphocytes (CTL) but it is difficult to eliminate allo-reactive CTLs and this treatment may cause graft versus host disease (GvHD), in which the patient's own normal cells are damaged or killed.

Strikingly, in sub-Saharan Africa, in the 'lymphoma belt', this typically leads to Burkitt's lymphoma, presenting most commonly as bilateral jaw tumours[32], this may be referred to as endemic or African Burkitt's. In other geographical locations BL may occur but in different anatomical sites, or other malignancies, including HL, may be seen.

The fundamental transforming event in BL is a translocation bringing the MYC oncogene under control of an immunoglobulin gene, leading to constitutive expression of MYC[32]. It was long accepted that a key cofactor in African BL was chronic malarial infection leading to immunosuppression. More recently, it has been suggested that there may be multiple cofactors contributing to this process[30].

Differing clinical presentations of EBV-associated malignancy in immunosuppressed individuals may reflect the influences of different cofactors, or they may indicate that different populations of B-cells have become transformed; in the case of EBV-associated Hodgkin lymphoma (HL), it appears that a key stage is abortive infection of germinal-centre B-cells in lymph nodes[5].

High incidence of EBV-associated NPC in Cantonese men is thought to reflect both genetic susceptibility and the high dietary intake of salted fish, which is a known risk factor for NPC[48]. Similar combinations of dietary, infectious and possibly genetic, risk factors are seen in Tunisia, which is another NPC high-risk area[49]. In the UK, in 2004, there were just 223 cases of nasopharyngeal cancer[50], with almost all cases seen in the UK occurring in the ethnic Chinese community[51].

Prevention

For over 30 years there has been discussion of the value of an EBV vaccine[52], yet none is available. The global ubiquity of the virus suggests that eradication would be a very difficult challenge. Given that most people in the developed world carry EBV with no ill-effects there is little incentive to take on such a colossal task[53]. In the developing world, where EBV morbidity and mortality are greatest, so too would be the logistical problems in delivering a vaccine.

In Africa, concentrating resources on eradication of malaria, a co-carcinogen for Burkitt lymphoma, would be markedly more cost-effective, given the economic burden of malarial infection[54]. Similarly, it would be far more economic, and probably more successful to educate Cantonese men on the hazards of salted fish than attempting to eradicate EBV in this population.

Kaposi sarcoma-associated herpesvirus (KSHV)/ human herpesvirus 8 (HHV-8)

Organism[55]

A gammaherpesvirus, with a double-stranded DNA genome variously reported as between 170 and 270kKb, which encodes for 75 genes, the virus persists in latently infected cells as a circular episome.

HHV-8 is the only human herpesvirus which is not ubiquitous in human populations; it has a geographically restricted distribution – *'the virus is prevalent in Africa, in Mediterranean countries, among Jews and Arabs and certain Amerindians'*[56]. In Uganda more than 80% of the population is HHV-8 positive[57]. Although different regions have different strains, these have not been shown to have differences in pathogenesis. HHV-8 is found more commonly and at higher levels in saliva than in other body fluids[58]; initially, it was believed that the virus was only transmitted sexually, but it is *'now also considered transmissible through low risk or more casual behaviors'*[59]. Although it is not thought to be transmitted vertically during the perinatal period, horizontal asexual transmission has been reported within families, probably by infected saliva[60]. Writing in 2005, Edelman stated, '*transmission via blood is possible, albeit with difficulty*'[59], although he went on to say, '*Larger studies are required to determine if HHV-8 is a true threat to the blood supply*'. Almost exactly a year later a study was published which showed that HHV-8 can be transmitted by transfusion[61]; the authors suggested that certain factors had made this study optimal for detecting transmission – '*a large study population, high seroprevalence of HHV-8 in the community, short duration of blood storage before transfusion, and absence of leukocyte reduction*' – the study had shown a significantly higher risk of transmission when blood was given after less than 4 days in storage. A recent report[62] indicated that '*transmission routes of HHV-8 differ strikingly between high- and low-prevalence areas*', although there is no adequate explanation for the difference; the report concludes that in the developed world any transmission risk is so low as not to warrant specific safety measures.

Solid organ transplant recipients have a significant risk of developing KS[63]; the degree of increased risk is largely dependent on the background level of HHV-8 positivity in the local population. Although HHV-8 can be transmitted within a solid organ from an infected donor[64], studies suggest that, certainly in areas of high incidence of HHV-8 infection, most KS in transplant recipients is due to reactivation of pre-existing host infection[65].

IARC status

Group 1 – definite carcinogen in humans[8].

Associated malignancies

HHV-8 has been causally linked to three distinct neoplasms, Kaposi sarcoma (KS), primary effusion lymphoma (PEL) and plasmablastic multi-centric Castleman's disease (MCD); for KS and PEL it is considered necessary but not sufficient, whereas MCD is often HHV-8 negative, especially in HIV-negative patients[59].

Kaposi sarcoma

By far the commonest malignancy associated with HHV-8 infection is Kaposi sarcoma; HHV-8 is considered a necessary, but not sufficient cause of KS[66]. '*The link between Kaposi's sarcoma and HHV-8 infection is especially relevant in sub-Saharan Africa, where Kaposi's sarcoma is now the most common malignancy in many countries*'[57]. A high incidence of KS in previously unaffected populations was one of the bellwethers which led to the recognition of AIDS[67]; initially a marked rise in incidence of KS was seen in Western countries, almost all in those with clinical AIDS, but the introduction of highly active antiretroviral therapy (HAART) has seen this reduce in recent years[68]. Cases of classic KS are now heavily outnumbered by HIV-associated cases (see Chapter 2 for a description of different forms of KS).

Primary effusion lymphoma

Primary effusion lymphoma (PEL) is a rare form of lymphoma with a unique clinical presentation, arising in body cavities such as the pleura, pericardium or peritoneum[69]. HHV-8 positivity is, by definition, a feature of PEL; the oncogenic pathways involved are unclear but the typical presentation is in an HIV-positive male[70], it has been suggested that HIV-negative cases may represent a distinct clinical entity[71]. About 90% of PEL cases are also positive for EBV but, as with HIV, the role of co-infection is unclear; intriguingly EBV-positive PEL cells all show hallmarks of having passed through lymph-node germinal centres (a stage in maturation of B-cells), whereas EBV-negative PEL cells may be either germinal centre/post-germinal centre or naive[72] – the significance of this is unknown. PEL is exceptionally rare in the HIV-negative population; when it does occur it affects the same populations prone to 'classic' KS, suggesting shared risk factors[73]. Even in the HIV-positive population, PEL is rare, being variously reported as making up only about 0.13%[70] to about 4% of AIDS-related non-Hodgkin lymphoma[74].

Plasmablastic multi-centric Castleman's disease

More commonly referred to simply as multi-centric Castleman's disease (MCD), this is a *'rare polyclonal B-cell angiolymphoproliferative disorder'*[59]. More than 90% of AIDS-associated cases of MCD are HHV-8 positive against around 40% of non-AIDS cases[75]. MCD is polyclonal and very variable in its presentation; although it is sometimes listed amongst cancers caused by HHV-8, other authors consider it be non-malignant[73]. In light of its rarity and the questions over whether it is a cancer, it will not be discussed further.

Unsubstantiated reports

Other malignancies have been suggested as being caused by HHV-8, most notably multiple myeloma.

Multiple myeloma

HHV-8 has been proposed as a causal factor for multiple myeloma[76]; studies in France[77] and the UK[78] have found no evidence of an association.

Cofactors

HIV infection appears to act as a cofactor to HHV-8 in both KS and PEL. Although both conditions are seen in HIV-naive patients, they are much more commonly seen as AIDS-defining lesions. It is unclear whether this reflects more than just the increased vulnerability of any immunosuppressed person to HHV 8-associated malignancies. A strong indication that there are other, yet unidentified, cofactors is the striking excess of KS in gay males compared with other HIV-positive populations such as haemophiliac children[55]. It is probable that there are also cofactors present in most cases of PEL, as this often occurs following KS and shows similar distribution – the rarity of PEL compared with KS makes it more difficult to identify specific cofactors.

Prevention

Although the modes of transmission of HHV-8 are not fully understood, it is thought that the most common is exposure in early life to infected saliva of a family member. In areas with the highest population prevalence of HHV-8, screening of blood donations for HHV-8 is not economically feasible and extended storage of blood prior to use has been shown to be associated with a high risk of bacterial infection[79]. 'WHO recommends that, at a minimum, blood be screened for HIV, hepatitis B, hepatitis C, and syphilis'[80]; yet, of 40 countries in sub-Saharan Africa for which data is available, 28 have been unable to meet this minimal screening level, so it is highly unlikely that HHV-8 screening will be feasible. A 2006 conference report[81] stated 'Nowhere in the world do blood transfusion services screen for HHV-8'; the authors reported that, in Uganda, there was a significantly higher death rate in those transfused with HHV-8 positive blood compared with those who received HHV-8 negative blood. The authors pointed out that it was not possible to exclude confounding due to other pathogens; this does raise the question whether developed countries should screen donations for HHV-8. Both the studies showing transfusion transmission and the study showing increased mortality took place in sub-Saharan African populations and thus cannot be taken as reliably predicting outcomes in developed world populations. There is clear evidence that HHV-8 related morbidity is higher in immunosuppressed populations but it is already routine practice for immunosuppressed patients to receive leukodepleted transfusions (which greatly reduce the scope for transmission of intracellular viruses such as HHV-8); it is strongly arguable that there is no need for any further measures in developed countries. Between 1995 and 2005 the cost of providing blood products in the UK roughly doubled, reaching £500 million, the increase was 'mainly due to newer anti-microbial tests and processes'[82]. The low level of infection in the donor population, low risk of transmission and low morbidity from HHV-8 mean that it is unlikely that routine screening would be deemed cost-effective in the UK; it may be of value to screen units being given to immunosuppressed patients.

There is currently no vaccine available against HHV-8; the impact of KS in the developed world is not sufficiently great to make this a priority, while in sub-Saharan Africa, where the problem is greatest, effective measures against HIV infection might be more effective, and would offer further benefit of preventing spread of HIV and of other STIs. In the developed world the introduction of HAART has greatly reduced the incidence of AIDS-related cancer[83].

There is clear evidence, unsurprisingly, that organ-transplant recipients are at increased risk of Kaposi sarcoma (KS) (and other immunodeficiency-associated malignancies). A study of US transplant recipients found that 8.8%

of almost 1/4 million patients developed KS[84]; risk factors were age, sex and citizenship status, which the authors suggest are indicators of the probability of pre-transplant HHV-8 status. It remains controversial whether transplanted organs are a significant vector of HHV-8 infection in previously naïve individuals.

Summary

■ Herpesviruses are ubiquitous in human and animal populations
  o More than 100 known types, grouped in three classes – α, β and γ
  o Eight are specific to humans – human herpesviruses (HHV)
■ Enveloped – large double-stranded DNA genome
■ Establish lifelong latency
  o May be reactivated especially in immunosuppressed host
■ All except HHV-7 have at least one known disease association
■ IARC designation
  o EBV and HHV-8 Group 1 (definite human carcinogens)
  o EBV is causally linked with many malignancies, most notably Burkitt's lymphoma and Hodgkin's lymphoma
  o KSV is causally linked with Kaposi's sarcoma, primary effusion lymphoma and multi-centric Castleman's disease
■ HHV-2 (HSV-2) is a cofactor with HPV in cervical cancer[2]

Herpesviruses are ubiquitous DNA viruses, causally linked with several different malignancies. For KS and PEL, it is thought that HHV-8 is a necessary but not sufficient causal factor. EBV shows a more complex relationship with BL and HL. Both BL and HL are heterogeneous conditions and it is thought that a proportion of cases of each are EBV related but that EBV is neither a necessary, nor a sufficient cause. EBV is a necessary but not sufficient causal agent for African endemic BL; in the developed world EBV-related BL is seen only in immunosuppressed populations. It is thought that there may be another, as yet unidentified, infectious trigger for HL.

Although there has been discussion on the feasibility of a vaccine against EBV, the ubiquity of the infection would make it a daunting task to achieve effective levels of herd immunity. It may be more realistic to address the cofactors of endemic BL, especially given the global impact of malaria – the most significant of these cofactors.

References

1. Timbury, M.C. & Edmond, E. (1979) Herpesviruses. *Journal of Clinical Pathology*, **32**, 859–881.
2. Smith, J.S., Herrero, R., Bosetti, C., *et al.* (2002) Herpes simplex virus-2 as a human papillomavirus cofactor in the etiology of invasive cervical cancer. *Journal of the National Cancer Institute*, **94**, 1604–1613.

3. Barton, E.S., White, D.W., Cathelyn, J.S., *et al.* (2007) Herpesvirus latency confers symbiotic protection from bacterial infection. *Nature*, **447**, 326–330.

4. Gallagher, A., Perry, J., Shield, L., Freeland, J., MacKenzie, J. & Jarrett, R.F. (2002) Viruses and Hodgkin disease: No evidence of novel herpesviruses in non-EBV-associated lesions. *International Journal of Cancer*, **101**, 259–264.

5. Young, L.S. & Rickinson, A.B. (2004) Epstein-Barr virus: 40 years on. *Nature Reviews Cancer*, **4**, 757–768.

6. Kuper, H., Adami, H.O. & Trichopolous, D. (2000) Infections as a major preventable cause of human cancer. *Journal of Internal Medicine*, **248**, 171–183.

7. Young, L.S. & Murray, P.G. (2003) Epstein-Barr virus and oncogenesis: From latent genes to tumours. *Oncogene*, **22**, 5108–5121.

8. IARC (1997) Epstein-Barr virus and Kaposi's sarcoma herpesvirus/human herpesvirus 8. *IARC Monographs on the Evaluation of Carcinogenic Risks to Humans*, **70**, 47.

9. Thompson, M.P. & Kurzrock, R. (2004) Epstein-Barr virus and cancer. *Clinical Cancer Research*, **10**, 803–821.

10. Carbone, A., Gloghini, A. & Dotti, G. (2008) EBV-associated lymphoproliferative disorders: Classification and treatment. *Oncologist*, **13**, 577–585.

11. Stewart, B.W. & Kleihues, P. (eds) (2003) The causes of cancer. In: *World Cancer Report*, Chap. 2, 120–81, pp. IARC Press Lyon, France.

12. IARC (1997) Epstein-Barr virus and Kaposi's sarcoma herpesvirus/human herpesvirus 8. *IARC Monographs on the Evaluation of Carcinogenic Risks to Humans*, **70**, 375.

13. Kuppers, R. (2009) The biology of Hodgkin's lymphoma. *Nature Reviews Cancer*, **9**, 15–27.

14. Kapatai, G. & Murray, P. (2007) Contribution of the Epstein Barr virus to the molecular pathogenesis of Hodgkin lymphoma. *Journal of Clinical Pathology*, **60**, 1342–1349.

15. Allemani, C., Sant, M., De Angelis, R., Marcos-Gragera, R. & Coebergh, J.W. (2006) Hodgkin disease survival in Europe and the U.S.: Prognostic significance of morphologic groups. *Cancer*, **107**, 352–360.

16. Ansell, S.M. & Armitage, J.O. (2006) Management of Hodgkin lymphoma. *Mayo Clinic Proceedings*, **81**, 419–426.

17. Re, D., Thomas, R.K., Behringer, K. & Diehl, V. (2005) From Hodgkin disease to Hodgkin lymphoma: Biologic insights and therapeutic potential. *Blood*, **105**, 4553–4560.

18. Jarrett, R.F., Krajewski, A.S., Angus, B., *et al.* (2003) The Scotland and Newcastle epidemiological study of Hodgkin's disease: Impact of histopathological review and EBV status on incidence estimates. *Journal of Clinical Pathology*, **56**, 811–816.

19. Andersson, J. (2006) Epstein-Barr virus and Hodgkin's lymphoma. *Herpes*, **13**, 12–16.

20. Jarrett, R.F. (2006) Viruses and lymphoma/leukaemia. *Journal of Pathology*, **208**, 176–186.

21. Kutok, J.L. & Wang, F. (2006) Spectrum of Epstein-Barr virus-associated diseases. *Annual Review of Pathology*, **1**, 375–404.

22. Nakatsuka, S. & Aozasa, K. (2006) Epidemiology and pathologic features of Hodgkin lymphoma. *International Journal of Hematology*, **83**, 391–397.

23. Tsang, R.W., Hodgson, D.C. & Crump, M. (2006) Hodgkin's lymphoma. *Current Problems in Cancer*, **30**, 107–158.

24. Tzankov, A. & Dirnhofer, S. (2006) Pathobiology of classical Hodgkin lymphoma. *Pathobiology*, **73**, 107–125.

25. Aldoss, I.T., Weisenburger, D.D., Fu, K., *et al.* (2008) Adult Burkitt lymphoma: Advances in diagnosis and treatment. *Oncology (Williston Park)*, **22**, 1508–1517.

26. Brady, G., Macarthur, G.J. & Farrell, P.J. (2008) Epstein-Barr virus and Burkitt lymphoma. *Postgraduate Medical Journal*, **84**, 372–377.

27. Thorley-Lawson, D.A. & Allday, M.J. (2008) The curious case of the tumour virus: 50 years of Burkitt's lymphoma. *Nature Reviews Microbiology*, **6**, 913–924.

28. Yustein, J.T. & Dang, C.V. (2007) Biology and treatment of Burkitt's lymphoma. *Current Opinion in Hematology*, **14**, 375–381.

29. Ferry, J.A. (2006) Burkitt's lymphoma: Clinicopathologic features and differential diagnosis. *Oncologist*, **11**, 375–383.

30. van den Bosch, C.A. (2004) Is endemic Burkitt's lymphoma an alliance between three infections and a tumour promoter? *Lancet Oncology*, **5**, 738–746.

31. Rochford, R., Cannon, M.J. & Moormann, A.M. (2005) Endemic Burkitt's lymphoma: A polymicrobial disease? *Nature Reviews Microbiology*, **3**, 182–187.

32. Brady, G., MacArthur, G.J. & Farrell, P.J. (2007) Epstein-Barr virus and Burkitt lymphoma. *Journal of Clinical Pathology*, **60**, 1397–1402.

33. Okano, M. & Gross, T.G. (2001) From Burkitt's lymphoma to chronic active Epstein-Barr virus (EBV) infection: An expanding spectrum of EBV-associated diseases. *Pediatric Hematology Oncology*, **18**, 427–442.

34. Ojha, J., Islam, N., Cohen, D.M., Marshal, D., Reavis, M.R. & Bhattacharyya, I. (2008) Post-transplant lymphoproliferative disorders of oral cavity. *Oral Surgery, Oral Medicine, Oral Pathology, Oral Radiology, and Endodontics*, **105**, 589–596.

35. Bakker, N.A. & van Imhoff, G.W. (2007) Post-transplant lymphoproliferative disorders: From treatment to early detection and prevention? *Haematologica*, **92**, 1447–1450.

36. Bakker, N.A., van Imhoff, G.W., Verschuuren, E.A. & van Son, W.J. (2007) Presentation and early detection of post-transplant lymphoproliferative disorder after solid organ transplantation. *Transplant International*, **20**, 207–218.

37. Zafar, S.Y., Howell, D.N. & Gockerman, J.P. (2008) Malignancy after solid organ transplantation: An overview. *Oncologist*, **13**, 769–778.

38. Dolcetti, R. (2007) B lymphocytes and Epstein-Barr virus: The lesson of post-transplant lymphoproliferative disorders. *Autoimmunity Reviews*, **7**, 96–101.

39. Aucejo, F., Rofaiel, G. & Miller, C. (2006) Who is at risk for post-transplant lymphoproliferative disorders (PTLD) after liver transplantation? *Journal of Hepatology*, **44**, 19–23.

40. Burney, K., Bradley, M., Buckley, A., Lyburn, I., Rye, A. & Hopkins, R. (2006) Posttransplant lymphoproliferative disorder: A pictorial review. *Australasian Radiology*, **50**, 412–418.

41. LaCasce, A.S. (2006) Post-transplant lymphoproliferative disorders. *Oncologist*, **11**, 674–680.

42. Lim, W.H., Russ, G.R. & Coates, P.T. (2006) Review of Epstein-Barr virus and post-transplant lymphoproliferative disorder post-solid organ transplantation. *Nephrology (Carlton)*, **11**, 355–366.

43. Mourad, W.A., Tulabah, A., Al Sayed, A., *et al.* (2006) The impact of the World Health Organization classification and clonality assessment of posttransplant lymphoproliferative disorders on disease management. *Archives of Pathology & Laboratory Medicine*, **130**, 1649–1653.

44. Perkins, J.D. (2006) Treatment strategies for posttransplant lymphoproliferative disorder. *Liver Transplantation*, **12**, 1013–1014.

45. Timuragaoglu, A., Ugur-Bilgin, A., Colak, D., *et al.* (2006) Posttransplant lymphoproliferative disorders in transplant recipients. *Transplantation Proceedings*, **38**, 641–645.

46. Trappe, R., Oertel, S. & Riess, H. (2006) Pathogenetic, clinical, diagnostic and therapeutic aspects of post-transplantation lymphoproliferative disorders. *Deutsches Aerzteblatt*, **103**, 3259–3267.

47. Lopes, V., Young, L.S. & Murray, P.G. (2003) Epstein-Barr virus-associated cancers: Aetiology and treatment. *Herpes*, **10**, 78–82.

48. Yu, M.C., Ho, J.H., Lai, S.H. & Henderson, B.E. (1986) Cantonese-style salted fish as a cause of nasopharyngeal carcinoma: Report of a case-control study in Hong Kong. *Cancer Research*, **46**, 956–961.

49. Jeannel, D., Hubert, A., de Vathaire, F., *et al.* (1990) Diet, living conditions and nasopharyngeal carcinoma in Tunisia – A case-control study. *International Journal of Cancer*, **46**, 421–425.

50. Toms, J.R. (2004) *CancerStats Monograph 2004: Cancer Incidence, Survival and Mortality in the UK and EU*. Cancer Research UK, London.

51. Warnakulasuricya, K.A., Johnson, N.W., Linklater, K.M. & Bell, J. (1999) Cancer of mouth, pharynx and nasopharynx in Asian and Chinese immigrants resident in Thames regions. *Oral Oncology*, **35**, 471–475.

52. Epstein, M.A. (1976) Implications of a vaccine for the prevention of Epstein-Barr virus infection: Ethical and logistic considerations. *Cancer Research*, **36**, 711–714.

53. de The, G. (1976) Epstein-Barr virus behavior in different populations and implications for control of Epstein-Barr virus-associated tumors. *Cancer Research*, **36**, 692–695.

54. Malaria no More and McKinsey & Co (2008) *We Can't Afford to Wait: The Business Case for Rapid Scale-up of Malaria Control in Africa*. Roll Back Malaria Partnership, Geneva, Switzerland.

55. Szajerka, T. & Jablecki, J. (2007) Kaposi's sarcoma revisited. *AIDS Reviews*, **9**, 3–10.

56. Boshoff, C. & Weiss, R.A. (2001) Epidemiology and pathogenesis of Kaposi's sarcoma-associated herpesvirus. *Philosophical Transactions of the Royal Society of London*, **356**, 517–534.

57. Senior, K. (2008) Kaposi's sarcoma: The persistent opportunist. *Lancet Oncology*, **9**, 705.

58. Pauk, J., Huang, M.L., Brodie, S.J., *et al.* (2000) Mucosal shedding of human herpesvirus 8 in men. *New England Journal of Medicine*, **343**, 1369–1377.

59. Edelman, D.C. (2005) Human herpesvirus 8 – A novel human pathogen. *Virology Journal*, **2**, 78.

60. Plancoulaine, S., Abel, L., van Beveren, M., *et al.* (2000) Human herpesvirus 8 transmission from mother to child and between siblings in an endemic population. *Lancet*, **356**, 1062–1065.

61. Hladik, W., Dollard, S.C., Mermin, J., *et al.* (2006) Transmission of human herpesvirus 8 by blood transfusion. *New England Journal of Medicine*, **355**, 1331–1338.

62. Vamvakas, E.C. (2010) Is human herpesvirus-8 transmitted by transfusion? *Transfusion Medicine Reviews*, **24**, 1–14.

63. Penn, I. (1979) Kaposi's sarcoma in organ transplant recipients: Report of 20 cases. *Transplantation*, **27**, 8–11.

64. Regamey, N., Tamm, M., Wernli, M., *et al.* (1998) Transmission of human herpesvirus 8 infection from renal-transplant donors to recipients. *New England Journal of Medicine*, **339**, 1358–1363.

65. Cattani, P., Capuano, M., Graffeo, R., *et al.* (2001) Kaposi's sarcoma associated with previous human herpesvirus 8 infection in kidney transplant recipients. *Journal of Clinical Microbiology*, **39**, 506–508.

66. Schwartz, R.A., Micali, G., Nasca, M.R. & Scuderi, L. (2008) Kaposi sarcoma: A continuing conundrum. *Journal of American Academy of Dermatology*, **59**, 179–206.

67. Friedman-Kien, A., Laubenstein, L., Marmor, M., *et al.* (1981) Kaposi's sarcoma and *Pneumocystis carinii* pneumonia among homosexual men – New York and California. *Morbidity and Mortality Weekly Report*, **30**, 250–252.

68. Horenstein, M.G., Moontasri, N.J. & Cesarman, E. (2008) The pathobiology of Kaposi's sarcoma: Advances since the onset of the AIDS epidemic. *Journal of Cutaneous Pathology*, **35** (Suppl. 2), 40–44.

69. Chen, Y.-B., Rahemtullah, A. & Hochberg, E. (2007) Primary effusion lymphoma. *Oncologist*, **12**, 569–576.

70. Mbulaiteye, S.M., Biggar, R.J., Goedert, J.J. & Engels, E.A. (2002) Pleural and peritoneal lymphoma among people with AIDS in the United States. *Journal of Acquired Immune Deficiency Syndromes*, **29**, 418–421.

71. Ascoli, V., Lo Coco, F., Torelli, G., *et al.* (2002) Human herpesvirus 8-associated primary effusion lymphoma in HIV- patients: A clinicoepidemiologic variant resembling classic Kaposi's sarcoma. *Haematologica*, **87**, 339–343.

72. Hamoudi, R., Diss, T.C., Oksenhendler, E., *et al.* (2004) Distinct cellular origins of primary effusion lymphoma with and without EBV infection. *Leukemia Research*, **28**, 333–338.

73. Sarid, R., Klepfish, A. & Schattner, A. (2002) Virology, pathogenetic mechanisms, and associated diseases of Kaposi sarcoma-associated herpesvirus (human herpesvirus 8). *Mayo Clinic Proceedings*, **77**, 941–949.

74. Simonelli, C., Spina, M., Cinelli, R., *et al.* (2003) Clinical features and outcome of primary effusion lymphoma in HIV-infected patients: A single-institution study. *Journal of Clinical Oncology*, **21**, 3948–3954.

75. Soulier, J., Grollet, L., Oksenhendler, E., *et al.* (1995) Kaposi's sarcoma-associated herpesvirus-like DNA sequences in multicentric Castleman's disease. *Blood*, **86**, 1276–1280.

76. Sjak-Shie, N.N., Vescio, R.A. & Berenson, J.R. (1999) The role of human herpesvirus-8 in the pathogenesis of multiple myeloma. *Hematology/Oncology Clinics of North America*, **13**, 1159–1167.

77. Cacoub, P., Ravaud, P., Calvez, V., Dupin, N., Bouscary, D. & Bossi, P. (1997) HHV-8 and multiple myeloma in France. *Lancet*, **350**, 1144.

78. MacKenzie, J., Sheldon, J., Morgan, G., Cook, G., Schulz, T.F. & Jarrett, R.F. (1997) HHV-8 and multiple myeloma in the UK. *Lancet*, **350**, 1144–1145.

79. Offner, P.J. (2004) Age of blood: Does it make a difference? *Critical Care*, **8**, S24–S26.

80. Anon (2007) Improving blood safety worldwide. *Lancet*, **370**, 361.

81. Hladik, W., Pellen, P., Downing, R., *et al.* (2006) Risk of death following transfusion of human herpesvirus 8-seropositive blood. In: *13th Conference on Retroviruses and Opportunistic Infection*, Denver, Colorado, 5–8 February 2006.

82. McClelland, D.B.I. & Contreras, M. (2005) Effectiveness and safety of blood transfusion: Have we lost the plot? *Journal of the Royal College of Physicians of Edinburgh*, **35**, 2–4.

83. Biggar, R.J., Chaturvedi, A.K., Goedert, J.J. & Engels, E.A. (2007) AIDS-related cancer and severity of immunosuppression in persons with AIDS. *Journal of National Cancer Institute*, **99**, 962–972.

84. Mbulaiteye, S.M. & Engels, E.A. (2006) Kaposi's sarcoma risk among transplant recipients in the United States (1993–2003). *International Journal of Cancer*, **119**, 2685–2691.

7 Hepatitis viruses

Viral infections of the liver are major risk factors for hepatocellular carcinoma, which is one of the five leading causes of cancer death globally[1]. Progress has been made with vaccination against hepatitis B, but much needs to be done to achieve optimum protection.

There are six human hepatitis viruses A, B, C, D, E and G[2]; of these, B and C are considered carcinogenic while D acts as a co-carcinogen. They differ in their mode of transmission, hepatitis B, C, D and G are transmitted by blood, or in body fluids, while hepatitis A and E are transmitted enterally. Thus, potentially carcinogenic hepatitis viruses can only be transmitted in body fluids; they are acquired perinatally, during sexual contact by IV drug users sharing paraphernalia or iatrogenically by therapeutic administration of blood or blood products. Hepatitis B is readily transmitted perinatally, while this is rarer for hepatitis C[3–5].

Hepatitis B (HBV) and hepatitis C (HCV) are in International Agency for Research on Cancer (IARC) Group 1 (definite human carcinogens) whereas hepatitis D is in Group 4 (not classifiable as to carcinogenicity in humans). Hepatitis D (HDV) is a 'satellite agent' to hepatitis B[6]; the HDV genome codes for a single protein, the HDV antigen and relies on HBV envelope proteins to form a virion. It can only form infectious particles when it invades a cell which is already infected with HBV. There is no specific vaccine or therapy against HDV, and studies suggest that, as would be expected, effective programmes targeting HBV infection can eliminate it. It will be discussed in this section as a cofactor for HBV-associated liver cancer, rather than as a separate entity; it is included on the basis of evidence suggesting that co-infection with HDV may exacerbate HBV-induced liver disease and thus increase the risk of malignant transformation.

Cirrhosis of the liver is a major risk factor for hepatocellular carcinoma (HCC); the highest incidence of malignant progression is seen in HCV-induced cirrhosis[7]. Hepatitis B is the major cause of HCC-related deaths worldwide, while increased incidence of hepatitis C in the US and Europe is fuelling an increased rate of HCC[7].

Hepatitis B has been referred to as a *'stealth virus'*[8] as it can establish a stable long-term infection without triggering an innate immune system response.

Infectious Causes of Cancer, first edition. By Ken Campbell. Published 2011 by John Wiley & Sons Ltd.
© 2011 John Wiley & Sons Ltd.

The adaptive (antibody-based) immune response is swamped by very large numbers of incomplete viral particles which 'mop-up' antibodies which may be produced[9,10]. In a proportion of cases the immune response is inadequate to clear the infection but triggers chronic subclinical inflammation leading to cirrhosis and potentially to hepatocellular carcinoma (HCC). Hepatitis C, in contrast, is highly immunogenic but *'cunningly evades the innate immune response and also defeats the adaptive immune response by mutation and functional inactivation'*[8]. For both HBV and HCV HCC typically occurs after 30 or more years of chronic infection[11]. A comparison of the proteomes of HCC cells associated with HBV and with HCV shows significant differences, supporting the hypothesis that there are distinct oncogenic pathways[12].

The other hepatitis viruses are hepatitis A and hepatitis E, which are transmitted enterically and hepatitis G which is transmitted parenterally, probably being both blood-borne and sexually transmitted; none of these is considered a carcinogen. A recent review[13] suggests that HGV hepatitis may not exist as a clinical entity – it explicitly states that *'investigators could not trace the clinical stages characteristic of HBV and HCV: acute hepatitis-chronic hepatitis-liver cirrhosis (LC)-hepatocellular carcinoma (HCC)'*. A 2008 review states that, *'Infection with HGV is common in the world'*, however *'the world food and drug administration considers it unnecessary to recommend donor blood to be tested for serum GBV-C RNA'*[13].

In 1970 the National Blood Service in the UK introduced screening of donated units for presence of HBV, this was followed by HCV testing in 1992 and the more sensitive nucleic acid test (NAT) for HCV in 1997[14]. It is now estimated that the risk per 100 000 units of transfusion transmitted HCV is no higher than 0.024 and that of HBV no greater than 0.176.

Hepatitis B[15]

IARC status

Hepatitis B (HBV) belongs to the hepadnavirus family of viruses, which are hepatotropic (selectively infect liver cells) and highly species-specific. HBV is the only hepadnavirus which infects humans although closely related species infect *'apes, woodchucks (woodchuck hepatitis virus [WHV]), squirrels (ground squirrel hepatitis virus [GSHV]), herons (heron hepatitis B virus), ducks (duck hepatitis B virus), geese (goose hepatitis B virus), and cranes (crane hepatitis B virus)'*[16]. Woodchuck and duck hepatitis viruses *'provide model systems for the study of viral replication, pathogenesis and evaluation of antiviral drugs against HBV'*[15]. Hepadnaviruses have a genome which is circular and partially double-stranded; this is transcribed to a single-stranded RNA from which reverse transcriptase generates fully double-stranded functional DNA. HBV mature virions exit the cell not by causing lysis but via the Golgi apparatus and endoplasmic reticulum; in other words by utilizing normal secretory processes; this is a significant factor in minimizing the immune reaction, although it is clearly not the only factor as HCV is also minimally cytopathic, yet provokes a strong innate immune reaction.

The HBV genome contains no known oncogenes; the HBx gene product is thought to play a key role in causation of HCC but its mode of action is unclear[15,16]. Transgenic mice expressing the HBx gene develop HCC[17]. Although integration of the HBV genome is a common precursor to HCC, evidence suggests that 'insertional mutagenesis' – in which integration activates an oncogene or inactivates a tumour suppressor – occurs rarely[18].

Chronic active infection leading to cirrhosis is a key risk factor for development of liver cancer. The outcome of HBV infection depends on the host's immune system; if the host immune response is adequate, the infection is rapidly and completely cleared, if the response is very weak, chronic inactive infection is established, with minimal liver damage. Chronic active hepatitis, potentially leading to cirrhosis, occurs when the host mounts an immune response which is inadequate to clear the infection, but which damages virus-infected liver cells[19,20]. As described in earlier chapters, an association between chronic inflammation and cancer is very well established. Although the majority of patients with HCC have pre-existing cirrhosis this is not a necessary factor for development of HBV-associated liver cancer, with up to 40% of the latter group developing HCC before cirrhosis[21].

Timing of infection is a critical determinant of the probability of chronic infection: 'Chronic infection occurs in approximately 90% of infected infants, 30% of infected children aged <5 years, and <5% of infected persons aged >5 years'[22]. This is highly significant for vaccination strategies as described below under prevention. In Africa and southern Asia, hepatitis B is predominantly acquired perinatally and is the principle cause of HCC; in the West, infection is more commonly acquired later in life and is less likely to become established as a chronic infection and thus less likely to lead to HCC[23]. HBV is transmitted by blood and body fluids; sexual transmission is common, especially among men having sex with men (MSM)[24]. The WHO has described HBV as second only to tobacco in importance as a carcinogen[25].

Hepatitis C[26]

IARC status

Group – 1 (definitely carcinogenic in humans)

Hepatitis C is an RNA virus, a member of the Flaviviridae family, which includes flaviviruses and pestiviruses. Like hepadnaviruses, there are a number of other species of flavivirus but only HCV infects humans and, conversely, humans are the only natural host for HCV[27]; related animal viruses have provided valuable model systems for research. The HCV genome is replicated in the cytoplasmic compartment; DNA integration of viral sequences does not occur, although changes are seen in the nucleoli of infected cells, the exact mechanisms involved remain unclear[28].

In countries and populations with low incidence of HBV infection, HCV infection is the principal cause of HCC[29]. There is no proven direct hepatocarcinogenic mechanism for HCV and it is thought that chronic inflammation is the most likely aetiology[23]. Co-infection with HBV and HCV has been reported to aggravate the severity of liver damage and accelerate development of HCC; it has been proposed that patients with HCV should be vaccinated against HBV[25]. A retrospective study of stored sera taken from US military recruits between 1948 and 1955 found a comparable incidence of HCV seropositivity to that of samples from military recruits and blood donors in the 1990s[30]; the same report concluded, on the basis of morbidity and mortality analysis that *'healthy HCV-positive persons may be at less risk for progressive liver disease than is currently thought'*. This belies reports of a striking increase in HCV infection between the 1960s and 1980s[31,32]; the explanation may lie in the fact that the reported increase is of clinical diagnoses of hepatitis while the report on military recruits indicated that overt disease in this young healthy group was uncommon.

The increase in the incidence of clinically overt HCV infection in the West was initially caused by transfusion-transmitted infection; latterly intravenous drug misuse is thought to be the principal route of spread[33,34]. As there is no vaccine currently available for HCV, the only intervention available to reduce spread is outreach programmes to educate drug users about risks and provide them with safe injecting equipment; limited successes of such schemes to date suggest that incidence of HCV-associated HCC will continue to rise in the West[35]. The long hiatus between infection and development of HCC has led epidemiologists to estimate that it will be at least 10–15 years before the transfusion-associated cases of HCC decline[36].

HCV is less specifically hepatotropic than HBV; it is also found in B lymphocyte populations[37]. There is considerable evidence to suggest that chronic HCV infection of lymphocytes leads to a condition called mixed cryoglobulinaemia, which in turn may lead to non-Hodgkin lymphoma (NHL)[38]. Although the evidence is less conclusive than for HCC, it is generally accepted that HCV infection may lead to B cell NHL. Some reports have indicated no, or at most very weak, links between HCV and NHL while others report a clear association; the explanation may lie with the marked regional variation, which in turn appears to relate to local levels of HCV infection[39].

HCV differs from HBV in that, although it is a blood-borne virus, sexual transmission is thought to occur rarely, if at all between heterosexual couples[40]; there is stronger evidence for sexual transmission in men who have sex with men[41,42].

In HCV positive donors the following possible transmission routes were identified[43] (in decreasing order of risk):

- Injection drug use
- Blood transfusion
- Sex with an intravenous drug user
- Having been in jail for more than 3 days
- Religious scarification
- Having been struck or cut with a bloody object

- Pierced ears or body parts
- Immunoglobulin injection

Evidence indicates that in developed countries HCV is a more common cause of HCC than HBV, whereas in the developing world the reverse is true[44].

Hepatitis D[45]

IARC status

Group – 4 (not classifiable as to carcinogenicity in humans).

Hepatitis D is a satellite virus to HBV; it is an incomplete virus and depends on the presence of functioning HBV in the same cell to be capable of forming a complete infective particle. Key points[46] about HDV are:

- It requires the presence of HBV to replicate
- It occurs only as co-infection or superinfection with HBV
- HDV infection cannot precede HBV infection
- HDV infection tends to increase severity of HBV infection but reduces the risk of carrier status
- Successful protective measures against HBV will reduce the incidence of HDV

Hepatitis D will not be discussed further in this chapter.

Associated malignancies

Hepatocellular carcinoma (HCC)[47,48]

Hepatocellular carcinoma (HCC) is the most common primary liver cancer, making up about 80% of cases. HCC is a major global public health concern; it is the third most common cause of cancer death in men and accounts for about 4% of all known cancers[49]. The incidence is higher in men than in women, ranking as fifth most common cancer in men and eighth most common in women. The incidence varies widely geographically, as does the identity of the viral cause – in the developing world HBV infection is the most common cause of HCC, whereas in Japan and in the Western world HCV is a more common cause.

About 25% of the global liver cancer incidence is due to HCV infection[50]. HCV is likely to become relatively more significant globally as a cause of HCC with the spread of HBV vaccination programmes; in the UK a Royal College of Physicians of Edinburgh report in 2004 stressed the urgent need to invest in resources to manage the likely increased impact of HCV on the NHS – they state *'What is certain is that, if we do not invest adequately now, we will not be able to afford the consequences of failing to tackle this epidemic'*[51].

In European populations, alcohol abuse is a major risk factor for cirrhosis and thus, potentially, for HCC. Alcohol and tobacco smoking both increase the risk of HCC in people with hepatitis virus infections[52]; alcohol is a risk factor for HCC even in those who are free of hepatitis virus infections, whereas tobacco is not. In African and South-East Asian populations stored food crops are commonly contaminated with the liver-specific carcinogen aflatoxin[53] – this is discussed further under cofactors and prevention.

Other malignancies

Hepatitis B and C viruses are both classified as definite human carcinogens by IARC, but this applies only to hepatocellular carcinoma (HCC). There are numerous reports of causal links between hepatitis C and other cancers but these are not (yet) recognized by IARC. Most recent reviews cite hepatitis C as a cause both of HCC and a proportion of cases of non-Hodgkin lymphoma (NHL). The evidence linking HCV with malignancies other than HCC is discussed below.

Lymphoproliferative disorders[54]

Hepatitis C has been implicated in the development of several lymphoproliferative disorders including mixed cryoglobulinaemia and B cell non-Hodgkin lymphoma (NHL)[39]. Other authors have challenged this proposition[55]. The level of association shows wide geographical variation; the strongest links are observed in areas with high background incidence of HCV infection. A meta-analysis of epidemiological studies concluded that, '*the fraction of NHL attributable to HCV infection would be upward of 10% in countries such as Italy, where 20% of NHL cases were found to be HCV positive. In countries where the prevalence of HCV seropositivity in the general population is very low (<1%), the proportion of NHL attributable to HCV infection would be less than 1%*'[56]; the meta-analysis probably reflects the consensus view. In practice it should be remembered that there may be sub-populations, such as current or past IV drug abusers, who are at relatively high risk of HCV-associated NHL; this is clinically significant since a patient who has HCV-initiated NHL may experience complete resolution of the NHL with effective treatment of the HCV infection[57]. In any patient presenting with extra-nodal NHL, who is from a high-risk group for hepatitis C infection, it would be reasonable to offer an initial course of antiviral treatment, as this may be sufficient to achieve resolution of the lymphoma.

The principle pathogenetic mechanism in HCV-associated NHL is thought to be chronic B cell stimulation, leading to proliferation with an increased risk of emergence of malignant B cell clones[58]. An additional mechanism appears to be virus-induced dysregulation of cellular signalling systems[59]. HCV-associated NHL are extra-nodal, typically affecting mucosa-associated lymphoid tissue (MALT)[60]. In the UK and in most of Western Europe they are thought to contribute little to the total burden of NHL.

Other malignancies tentatively associated with hepatitis C infection include:

■ Cholangiocarcinoma[61]
■ Plasma cell leukaemia[62]
■ Thyroid cancer[63]
■ Lichen planus[64]
■ Squamous cell carcinoma of head and neck[65]

The following conditions have been specifically reported as not associated with hepatitis C infection:

■ Mycosis fungoides[66]
■ Myeloid malignancy[67]
■ HIV-associated Kaposi sarcoma[68]
■ Waldenstrom's macroglobulinaemia[69]

Cofactors

The most common cofactors for HCC are alcohol consumption (in the developed world) and aflatoxin contamination of stored food (in the developing world). Co-infections with any combination of HBV/HCV/HIV also increase the risk of malignant transformation.

Alcohol

In an Italian study[52] it was found that increasing alcohol consumption showed a clearly synergistic effect. In the hepatitis virus negative group heavy drinkers had an HCC incidence almost 5 times those with a low alcohol intake. In the hepatitis virus positive group heavy drinkers had an HCC incidence 2.5 times greater than those with a low alcohol intake but their risk was almost 75 times that of those who were virus negative and light drinkers.

Aflatoxin[70]

Aflatoxin is the name given to any of a group of chemically related compounds produced by mould species of the genus *Aspergillus*, its name is derived from the name of one of these species – *Aspergillus flavus toxin*; this species having been widely used in early research on the toxins. There are several distinct but chemically related aflatoxins – the most commonly seen are:

■ Blue-fluorescing
  o B1
  o B2

- Green-fluorescing
  - o G1
  - o G2
- Milk/meat forms
  - o M1
  - o M2

Aflatoxin B1 is the most common form; B2, G1 and G2 are generally not seen in the absence of G1. The M forms are found in milk, milk products and meat (hence M); they are formed by hydroxylation of B1 and B2 forms after an animal has ingested these. *A. flavus*, which occurs globally, produces aflatoxins B1 and B2; *A. parasiticus* occurs principally in the Americas and Africa, and produces B1, B2, G1 and G2 aflatoxins.

Aflatoxin-producing mould species may grow on plants in the field but are more commonly found on improperly stored foodstuffs. Aflatoxins have been detected in many foodstuffs, particularly;

- Dairy products
  - o Milk
  - o Cheese
- Corn and other cereals
- Peanuts
- Cotton seed
- Nuts
- Figs

If animals have received aflatoxin-contaminated feed this may lead to milk and milk products, eggs and meat products being contaminated (generally with aflatoxins M1 and M2). In most parts of the world corn contamination is the most serious problem but local variations may occur – in West Africa peanut contamination is more significant.

Aflatoxin B1 is classified by IARC as Group 1 (definitely carcinogenic in humans); in the overwhelmingly majority of cases it appears to act as a cofactor to hepatitis B[71]. Invasive infection by *Aspergillus* is rare and almost exclusively seen in the context of severe immunosuppression. HCC is not associated with clinical *Aspergillus* infection so, in this context, *Aspergillus* infection cannot be classed as an infectious cause of cancer in humans.

Prevention

Virus infection

The principal scope for prevention of virus-induced HCC is by vaccination against HBV infection. This has already been shown to be effective in population level trials in Africa[72], Taiwan[73,74], Alaska[75] and Italy[76] among others. Successive UK governments have chosen not to implement universal HBV vaccination, electing instead to vaccinate only infants deemed to be high risk. The US first introduced HBV vaccination in 1982, extending this to include universal neonatal vaccination in 1991[77], in 1997 this was expanded to extend vaccination to all vulnerable children under 18 years old[78]. In 2004 the effect of the policy was reviewed and it was shown that between 1990 and 2002 the incidence had fallen by 67%, with many remaining cases being diagnosed in immigrants who had not been part of the programme[79,80]. A *BMJ* review[81] stated in 2004, '*The United Kingdom is one of the few developed countries that have not implemented universal neonatal hepatitis B immunisation*'; in 2007 a paper[82] asked the question '*Should hepatitis B vaccination be introduced into childhood immunisation programmes in northern Europe?*', the authors summarized by saying, '*In conclusion, we recommend that Denmark, Finland, Iceland, Ireland, the Netherlands, Norway, Sweden, and the UK reassess their current at-risk hepatitis B immunisation policy and consequent public-health strategy. Global hepatitis B universal vaccination is ultimately the only way to eliminate HBV transmission and new cases of hepatitis B*'.

No vaccine is currently available against hepatitis C; this means that protection currently depends on primary prevention, that is, measures to minimize the risk of transmission. In the developed world, screening of blood for transfusion has almost eliminated this as a risk factor; transmission is now principally by sharing of contaminated drug injection paraphernalia and maternal-infant. Campaigns to reduce transmission of blood-borne hepatitis C can also be expected to reduce transmission of other blood-borne virus diseases, including HIV/AIDS and other forms of hepatitis. They are, therefore, likely to be highly cost-effective; recent reviews have considered the cost-effectiveness of hepatitis C control in the US, Uganda and in the UK[83–85]. A 2006 *BMJ* review on hepatitis C[86] indicated that chronic Hep C infection is now the leading indication for liver transplantation in the developed world and that latent infection means that, even with effective action, the incidence will continue to rise for 10–20 years. Strategies which have been suggested to reduce transmission among injecting drug users include:

- Improving knowledge of healthcare workers on how to prevent substance misuse and treat users
- Programmes to teach users safe injection practice
- Wide availability of needle exchange programmes and clean syringes – unfortunately, the UK Prison Service continues to rule out needle exchange schemes within prisons on the grounds that this condones illegal drug use, even though it provides bleach for sterilizing drug paraphernalia
- Community-based programmes to support and educated users of injected drugs
- Improved coordination between medical, mental health and non-medical support services
- Express measures to reduce transmission within the prison system, especially improved access to counselling and healthcare

Alcohol

Alcohol harm reduction programmes are in place throughout the developed world. Excess alcohol intake has been associated with many clinical conditions. There are no liver cancer-specific campaigns. In February 2009, the Scottish Nationalist Party announced plans to make Scotland the first country in Europe to fix a minimum price on alcoholic drinks[87]. There are multiple justifications for alcohol control campaigns; liver damage is a significant one among these, but cancer resulting from alcohol-induced liver disease is a low absolute risk.

Aflatoxin[88]

Aflatoxin contributes little or nothing to risk in the developed world but is a major factor in much of the developed world. Strategies to reduce the risk should probably, at present, concentrate on protecting food from contamination during harvesting and storage. Simple and inexpensive measures can be highly effective:

■ Drying crops on mats in the sun
■ Visual inspection and discarding visibly mouldy kernels or nuts before storage
■ Use of natural fibre sacks for storage
■ Keeping storage sacks on wooden pallets to keep the crop dry

Although aflatoxin and hepatitis B infection appear to be highly synergistic, there is clear evidence that aflatoxins are genotoxic and it would be unsafe to assume that they are only carcinogenic in hepatitis virus-infected individuals[71]. For this reason, measures against aflatoxin contamination should be undertaken in all areas, not only where HBV infection is endemic.

Summary

■ There are six human hepatitis viruses A, B, C, D, E and G.
  ○ Two are considered carcinogenic (B and C) while D acts a co-carcinogen
■ Hepatitis B, C, D and G are transmitted by blood, or in body fluids
■ Hepatitis A and E are transmitted enterally
■ IARC designation
  ○ Hepatitis B and C – Group 1 (definite human carcinogens)
  ○ Hepatitis D – Group 4 (not classifiable)

Hepatitis virus-induced HCC is one of the major categories of infection-associated cancers. The impact of hepatitis B in the developed world has been reduced by the introduction of a vaccine; at present, there is no vaccine against hepatitis C, so control depends on primary prevention of infection. If diagnosed early, hepatitis C is often responsive to antiviral chemotherapy. Until a vaccine is available, it is likely that hepatitis C will continue to be the major infectious cause of HCC in the developed world; in the developing world, hepatitis B continues to be a significant problem.

References

1. Garcia, M., Jemal, A., Ward, E.M., *et al.* (2007) *Global Cancer Facts & Figures 2007*. American Cancer Society, Atlanta, Georgia.

2. Hall, G.F. (2007) Hepatitis A, B, C, D, E, G: An update. *Ethnic Discrimination*, **17**, S2–S5.

3. Tang, J.R., Hsu, H.Y., Lin, H.H., *et al.* (1998) Hepatitis B surface antigenemia at birth: A long-term follow-up study. *Journal of Pediatrics*, **133**, 374–377.

4. Resti, M., Azzari, C., Mannelli, F., *et al.* (1998) Mother to child transmission of hepatitis C virus: Prospective study of risk factors and timing of infection in children born to women seronegative for HIV-1. *BMJ*, **317**, 437–441.

5. Syriopoulou, V., Nikolopoulou, G., Daikos, G.L., *et al.* (2005) Mother to child transmission of hepatitis C virus: Rate of infection and risk factors. *Scandinavian Journal of Infectious Diseases*, **37**, 350–353.

6. IARC (1997) *Hepatitis viruses.* International Agency for Research on Cancer, Lyon, France.

7. Schuppan, D. & Afdhal, N.H. (2008) Liver cirrhosis. *Lancet*, **371**, 838–851.

8. Wieland, S.F. & Chisari, F.V. (2005) Stealth and cunning: Hepatitis B and hepatitis C viruses. *Journal of Virology*, **79**, 9369–9380.

9. Ganem, D. & Prince, A.M. (2004) Hepatitis B virus infection – Natural history and clinical consequences. *New England Journal of Medicine*, **350**, 1118–1129.

10. Goodsell, D.S. (2007) The molecular perspective: Hepatitis B virus. *Oncologist*, **12**, 516–517.

11. Tong, M.J., el-Farra, N.S., Reikes, A.R., *et al.* (1995) Clinical outcomes after transfusion-associated hepatitis C. *New England Journal of Medicine*, **332**, 1463–1466.

12. Kim, W., Lim, S.O., Kim, J.S., *et al.* (2003) Comparison of proteome between hepatitis B virus- and hepatitis C virus-associated hepatocellular carcinoma. *Clinical Cancer Research*, **9**, 5493–5500.

13. Reshetnyak, V.I., Karlovich, T.I. & Ilchenko, L.U. (2008) Hepatitis G virus. *World Journal of Gastroenterology*, **14**, 4725–4734.

14. McClelland, D.B.L. & Contreras, M. (2005) Effectiveness and safety of blood transfusion: Have we lost the plot? *Journal of the Royal College of Physicians of Edinburg*, **35**, 2–4.

15. Block, T.M., Guo, H. & Guo, J.T. (2007) Molecular virology of hepatitis B virus for clinicians. *Clinics in Liver Diseases*, **11**, 685–706.

16. Bouchard, M.J. & Schneider, R.J. (2004) The enigmatic X gene of hepatitis B virus. *Journal of Virology*, **78**, 12725–12734.

17. Cui, F., Wang, Y., Wang, J., *et al.* (2006) The up-regulation of proteasome subunits and lysosomal proteases in hepatocellular carcinomas of the HBx gene knockin transgenic mice. *Proteomics*, **6**, 498–504.

18. Lupberger, J. & Hildt, E. (2007) Hepatitis B virus-induced oncogenesis. *World Journal of Gastroenterology*, **13**, 74–81.

19. Guidotti, L.G. & Chisari, F.V. (2006) Immunobiology and pathogenesis of viral hepatitis. *Annual Review of Pathology*, **1**, 23–61.

20. Baumert, T.F., Thimme, R. & von Weizsacker, F. (2007) Pathogenesis of hepatitis B virus infection. *World Journal of Gastroenterology*, **13**, 82–90.

21. McGlynn, K.A. & London, W.T. (2005) Epidemiology and natural history of hepatocellular carcinoma. *Best Practice & Research Clinical Gastroenterology*, **19**, 3–23.

22. Mast, E.E., Margolis, H.S., Fiore, A.E., *et al.* (2005) A comprehensive immunization strategy to eliminate transmission of hepatitis B virus infection in the United States: Recommendations of the Advisory Committee on Immunization Practices (ACIP) part 1: Immunization of infants, children, and adolescents. *MMWR Recommendations and Reports*, **54**, 1–31.

23. Schwartz, M., Roayaie, S. & Konstadoulakis, M. (2007) Strategies for the management of hepatocellular carcinoma. *Nature Clinical Practice Oncology*, **4**, 424–432.

24. van Houdt, R., Bruisten, S.M., Koedijk, F.D., *et al.* (2007) Molecular epidemiology of acute hepatitis B in the Netherlands in 2004: Nationwide survey. *Journal of Medical Virology*, **79**, 895–901.

25. Gomaa, A.I., Khan, S.A., Toledano, M.B., Waked, I. & Taylor-Robinson, S.D. (2008) Hepatocellular carcinoma: Epidemiology, risk factors and pathogenesis. *World Journal of Gastroenterology*, **14**, 4300–4308.

26. Wong, T. & Lee, S.S. (2006) Hepatitis C: A review for primary care physicians. *Canadian Medical Association Journal*, **174**, 649–659.

27. Chevaliez, S. & Pawlotsky, J.M. (2007) Hepatitis C virus: Virology, diagnosis and management of antiviral therapy. *World Journal of Gastroenterology*, **13**, 2461–2466.

28. Falcon, V., Acosta-Rivero, N., Chinea, G., *et al.* (2003) Nuclear localization of nucleocapsid-like particles and HCV core protein in hepatocytes of a chronically HCV-infected patient. *Biochemical and Biophysical Research Communications*, **310**, 54–58.

29. McLaughlin-Drubin, M.E. & Munger, K. (2008) Viruses associated with human cancer. *Biochimica et Biophysica Acta*, **1782**, 127–150.

30. Seeff, L.B., Miller, R.N., Rabkin, C.S., *et al.* (2000) 45-year follow-up of hepatitis C virus infection in healthy young adults. *Annals of Internal Medicine*, **132**, 105–111.

31. Alter, M.J., Hadler, S.C., Judson, F.N., *et al.* (1990) Risk factors for acute non-A, non-B hepatitis in the United States and association with hepatitis C virus infection. *Journal of the American Medical Association*, **264**, 2231–2235.

32. Armstrong, G.L., Alter, M.J., McQuillan, G.M. & Margolis, H.S. (2000) The past incidence of hepatitis C virus infection implications for the future burden of chronic liver disease in the United States. *Hepatology*, **31**, 777–782.

33. Busch, M.P., Glynn, S.A., Stramer, S.L., *et al.* (2005) A new strategy for estimating risks of transfusion-transmitted viral infections based on rates of detection of recently infected donors. *Transfusion*, **45**, 254–264.

34. Hagan, H., Thiede, H., Weiss, N.S., Hopkins, S.G., Duchin, J.S. & Alexander, E.R. (2001) Sharing of drug preparation equipment as a risk factor for hepatitis C. *American Journal of Public Health*, **91**, 42–46.

35. Hagan, H., Campbell, J., Thiede, H., *et al.* (2006) Self-reported hepatitis C virus antibody status and risk behavior in young injectors. *Public Health Reports*, **121**, 710–719.

36. Trinchet, J.C., Ganne-Carrie, N., Nahon, P., N'kontchou, G. & Beaugrand, M. (2007) Hepatocellular carcinoma in patients with hepatitis C virus-related chronic liver disease. *World Journal of Gastroenterology*, **13**, 2455–2460.

37. Ferri, C., la Civita, L., Monti, M., *et al.* (1996) Chronic hepatitis C and B-cell non-Hodgkin's lymphoma. *QJM*, **89**, 117–122.

38. Ferri, C., Caracciolo, F., Zignego, A.L., *et al.* (1994) Hepatitis C virus infection in patients with non-Hodgkin's lymphoma. *British Journal of Haematology*, **88**, 392–394.

39. Mazzaro, C., Tirelli, U. & Pozzato, G. (2005) Hepatitis C virus and non-Hodgkin's lymphoma 10 years later. *Digestive Liver Disease*, **37**, 219–226.

40. McMahon, J.M., Pouget, E.R. & Tortu, S. (2007) Individual and couple-level risk factors for hepatitis C infection among heterosexual drug users: A multilevel dyadic analysis. *Journal of Infectious Diseases*, **195**, 1572–1581.

41. Danta, M., Brown, D., Bhagani, S., *et al.* (2007) Recent epidemic of acute hepatitis C virus in HIV-positive men who have sex with men linked to high-risk sexual behaviours. *AIDS*, **21**, 983–991.

42. van de Laar, T.J., van der Bij, A.K., Prins, M., *et al.* (2007) Increase in HCV incidence among men who have sex with men in Amsterdam most likely caused by sexual transmission. *Journal of Infectious Diseases*, **196**, 230–238.

43. Wasmuth, J.-C. (2009) Hepatitis C – Epidemiology, transmission and natural history. In: *Hepatology 2009* (eds S. Mauss, T. Berg, J. Rockstroh, C. Sarrazin & H. Wedemeyer), pp. 37–48. Flying Publisher, Dusseldorf.

44. Mustapha, S., Bolori, M., Ajayi, N., *et al.* (2007) Hepatitis C antibodies in Nigerians with hepatocellular carcinoma. *The Internet Journal of Oncology*, **4** (2). http://www.ispub.com/ostia/index. php?xmlFilePath=journals/ijo/vol4n2/hepatitis.xml (accessed 21 June 2010).

45. Taylor, J.M. (2006) Hepatitis delta virus. *Virology*, **344**, 71–76.

46. Tepper, M.L. & Gully, P.R. (1997) Viral hepatitis: Know your D, E, F, and Gs. *Canadian Medical Association Journal*, **156**, 1735–1736.

47. Abou-Alfa, G. (2006) Hepatocellular carcinoma: Molecular biology and therapy. *Seminars in Oncology*, **33**, S79–S83.

48. Hamilton, S.R. & Aaltonen, L.A. (2000) Tumours of the liver and intrahepatic bile ducts. In: *World Health Organization Classification of Tumours. Pathology and Genetics of Tumours of the Digestive System* (eds S.R. Hamilton & L.A. Aaltonen), pp. 157–202. International Agency for Research on Cancer, Lyon, France.

49. Stewart, B.W. & Kleihues, P. (2003) Human cancers by organ site. In: *World Cancer Report* (eds B.W. Stewart & P. Kleihues), pp. 181–270. International Agency for Research on Cancer, Lyon, France.

50. Alter, M.J. (2007) Epidemiology of hepatitis C virus infection. *World Journal of Gastroenterology*, **13**, 2436–2441.

51. Editorial – RCPE (2004) Consensus statement: Hepatitis C. *Journal of the Royal College of Physicians of Edinburgh*, **34**, 196–197.

52. Franceschi, S., Montella, M., Polesel, J., *et al.* (2009) Hepatitis viruses, alcohol, and tobacco in the etiology of hepatocellular carcinoma in Italy. *Cancer Epidemiology Biomarkers & Prevention*, **15**, 683–689.

53. Goldman, R. & Shields, P.G. (2003) Food mutagens. *Journal of Nutrition*, **133**, 965S–973S.

54. Libra, M., Gasparotto, D., Gloghini, A., Navolanic, P.M., De Re, V. & Carbone, A. (2005) Hepatitis C virus (HCV) infection and lymphoproliferative disorders. *Frontiers in Bioscience*, **10**, 2460–2471.

55. Aviles, A., Valdez, L., Halabe, J., *et al.* (2003) No association between lymphoma and hepatitis C virus. *Medical Oncology*, **20**, 165–168.

56. Dal Maso, L. & Franceschi, S. (2006) Hepatitis C virus and risk of lymphoma and other lymphoid neoplasms: A meta-analysis of epidemiologic studies. *Cancer Epidemiology Biomarkers & Prevention*, **15**, 2078–2085.

57. Kelaidi, C., Rollot, F., Park, S., *et al.* (2004) Response to antiviral treatment in hepatitis C virus-associated marginal zone lymphomas. *Leukemia*, **18**, 1711–1716.

58. Wiwanitkit, V. (2007) Hepatitis virus infection and Hodgkin's lymphoma: A review of the literature. *Hepatitis Monthly*, **7**, 229–231.

59. Landau, D.A., Saadoun, D., Calabrese, L.H. & Cacoub, P. (2007) The pathophysiology of HCV induced B-cell clonal disorders. *Autoimmunity Reviews*, **6**, 581–587.

60. Zucca, E., Roggero, E., Maggi-Solca, N., *et al.* (2000) Prevalence of *Helicobacter pylori* and hepatitis C virus infections among non-Hodgkin's lymphoma patients in Southern Switzerland. *Haematologica*, **85**, 147–153.

61. Okuda, K., Nakanuma, Y. & Miyazaki, M. (2002) Cholangiocarcinoma: Recent progress. Part 1: Epidemiology and etiology. *Journal of Gastroenterology and Hepatology*, **17**, 1049–1055.

62. Hermouet, S., Corre, I., Gassin, M., Bigot-Corbel, E., Sutton, C.A. & Casey, J.W. (2003) Hepatitis C virus, human herpesvirus 8, and the development of plasma-cell leukemia. *New England Journal of Medicine*, **348**, 178–179.

63. Montella, M., Pezzullo, L., Crispo, A., *et al.* (2003) Risk of thyroid cancer and high prevalence of hepatitis C virus. *Oncology Reports*, **10**, 133–136.

64. Nagao, Y. & Sata, M. (2004) Hepatitis C virus and lichen planus. *Journal of Gastroenterology and Hepatology*, **19**, 1101–1113.

65. Nobles, J., Wold, C., Fazekas-May, M., Gilbert, J. & Friedlander, P.L. (2004) Prevalence and epidemiology of hepatitis C virus in patients with squamous cell carcinoma of the head and neck. *Laryngoscope*, **114**, 2119–2122.

66. Miertusova, S., Bonin, S., Trevisan, G. & Stanta, G. (2004) Mycosis fungoides is not associated with hepatitis C virus infection. *British Journal of Dermatology*, **151**, 1108–1110.

67. Murashige, N., Kami, M., Iwata, H., Kishi, Y. & Matsuo, K. (2005) No relationship between hepatitis C infection and risk of myeloid malignancy. *Haematologica*, **90**, 572–574.

68. Schepers, K., Van Vooren, J.P. & Simonart, T. (2006) Hepatitis C virus is not a cofactor for Kaposi's sarcoma development in HIV-infected patients. *International Journal of Dermatology*, **45**, 994–995.

69. Leleu, X., O'Connor, K., Ho, A.W., *et al.* (2007) Hepatitis C viral infection is not associated with Waldenstrom's macroglobulinemia. *American Journal of Hematology*, **82**, 83–84.

70. Ritchie, J.C. (2007) Aflatoxin. In: *Molecules of Death* (eds R.H. Waring, G.B. Steventon & S.C. Mitchell), pp. 1–18. World Scientific Publishing Company Ltd, Singapore.

71. IARC (2002) Some traditional herbal medicines, some mycotoxins, naphthalene and styrene. *IARC Monographs on the Evaluation of Carcinogenic Risks to Humans*, **82**, 171–300.

72. Whittle, H., Jaffar, S., Wansbrough, M., *et al.* (2002) Observational study of vaccine efficacy 14 years after trial of hepatitis B vaccination in Gambian children. *BMJ*, **325**, 569.

73. Kane, M.A. (2003) Global control of primary hepatocellular carcinoma with hepatitis B vaccine: The contributions of research in Taiwan. *Cancer Epidemiology Biomarkers & Prevention*, **12**, 2–3.

74. Chemin, I. (2010) Evaluation of a hepatitis B vaccination program in Taiwan: Impact on hepatocellular carcinoma development. *Future Oncology*, **6**, 21–23.

75. McMahon, B.J., Bruden, D.L., Petersen, K.M., *et al.* (2005) Antibody levels and protection after hepatitis B vaccination: Results of a 15-year follow-up. *Annals of Internal Medicine*, **142**, 333–341.

76. Zanetti, A.R., Mariano, A., Romano, L., *et al.* (2005) Long-term immunogenicity of hepatitis B vaccination and policy for booster: An Italian multicentre study. *Lancet*, **366**, 1379–1384.

77. Hollinger, F.B. (1996) Comprehensive control (or elimination) of hepatitis B virus transmission in the United States. *Gut*, **38** (Suppl. 2), S24–S30.

78. Anon (1999) Update: Recommendations to prevent hepatitis B virus transmission – United States. *MMWR Morbidity and Mortality Weekly Report*, **48**, 33–34.

79. Anon (2004) Acute hepatitis B among children and adolescents–United States, 1990–2002. *MMWR Morbidity and Mortality Weekly Report*, **53**, 1015–1018.

80. Anon (2004) Incidence of acute hepatitis B–United States, 1990–2002. *MMWR Morbidity and Mortality Weekly Report*, **52**, 1252–1254.

81. Aggarwal, R. & Ranjan, P. (2004) Preventing and treating hepatitis B infection. *BMJ*, **329**, 1080–1086.

82. Zuckerman, J., van Hattum, J., Cafferkey, M., *et al.* (2007) Should hepatitis B vaccination be introduced into childhood immunisation programmes in northern Europe? *Lancet Infectious Diseases*, **7**, 410–419.

83. McHutchison, J.G., Bacon, B.R. & Owens, G.S. (2007) Making it happen: Managed care considerations in vanquishing hepatitis C. *American Journal of Managed Care*, **13** (Suppl. 12), quiz S337–340, S327–S336.

84. Hladik, W., Kataaha, P., Mermin, J., *et al.* (2006) Prevalence and screening costs of hepatitis C virus among Ugandan blood donors. *Tropical Medicine and International Health*, **11**, 951–954.

85. Shah, B.B. & Wong, J.B. (2006) The economics of hepatitis C virus. *Clinics in Liver Disease*, **10**, 717–734.

86. Patel, K., Muir, A.J. & McHutchison, J.G. (2006) Diagnosis and treatment of chronic hepatitis C infection. *BMJ*, **332**, 1013–1017.

87. Taylor, J. (3 March 2009) Scotland to end 'pocket money' prices for drink. *Independent*, **10**.

88. Hall, A.J. & Wild, C.P. (2003) Liver cancer in low and middle income countries. *BMJ*, **326**, 994–995.

8 Human papillomaviruses

Human papillomavirus (HPV) infection is geographically ubiquitous; individual rates of infection are so high that it has been suggested that 70–80% of all sexually active individuals will be infected at some point in their life[1]. If all types are included it is probable that all people are infected at some time. There are more than 100 subtypes distinguished on the basis of DNA sequence; over 40 strains are known to infect the human anogenital tract[2]. A minority of these are classed as International Agency for Research on Cancer (IARC) Group 1 – definite carcinogenic in humans HPV 16, 18, 31, 33, 35, 39, 45, 51, 52, 56, 58, 59, 66, HPV genus-beta types 5 and 8.

Rates of cervical cancer have been reduced in the developed world by programmes which screen for, and treat, pre-malignant lesions[3]. The introduction of HPV vaccine covering the most ubiquitous carcinogenic strains is expected to further reduce the incidence of HPV-related cancer in developed nations.

In the developing world, HPV-related cervical cancer is a leading cause of female cancer mortality; it has been estimated that in 2009 89% of new cases of cervical cancer will occur in the developing world[4]. HPV is also causally linked with cancer of the vulva, vagina, penis and anus, and with head and neck cancer (cancer of the oral cavity and oropharynx)[5]. The incidence of HPV-related head and neck cancer is reported to be correlated with oral sex, especially among young people; fortunately HPV-positive cases have been reported to have a good prognosis[6,7], although some (small) studies have shown no influence[8].

The organism[9–11]

Papillomaviruses are small DNA viruses with a circular single-stranded genome. The taxonomic classification of papillomaviruses has undergone marked revisions[12]. Papillomaviruses were originally included in a wider family called the papovaviruses[13]; it was only relatively recently that this was split into the polyomavirus and papillomavirus families, on the basis of significant differences, not least of which was the fact that they share very few common genetic sequences[5].

Infectious Causes of Cancer, first edition. By Ken Campbell. Published 2011 by John Wiley & Sons Ltd.
© 2011 John Wiley & Sons Ltd.

All papillomaviruses are abbreviated PV, with a prefix indicating the host species, thus all types which infect humans are classed as HPV[14]. There are over 100 different HPV types, classified on the basis of genetic sequence analysis. Human papillomaviruses are grouped into genera; around 90% of HPV strains belong to either the alpha or beta papillomavirus genera.

The alpha genus is most clinically important; it contains all the HPV types associated with mucosal and genital lesions, and therefore accounts for most HPV-associated malignancies. The alpha papillomaviruses include both high and low risk strains. Beta papillomaviruses are associated with cutaneous lesions, which are predominantly benign, but may be malignant in patients with epidermodysplasia verruciformis (EV) or who are immunosuppressed. Of the remaining genera (gamma to pi papillomavirus) only gamma and mu infect humans, and neither is considered carcinogenic in any patient population[14].

Taxonomy within HPV has a high clinical significance – a small number of high risk strains account for almost all cervical malignancies. HPV 16 and 18 are the most highly carcinogenic accounting for about 70% of cervical cancer, and about 50% of high-grade cervical intraepithelial neoplasia (CIN), which are pre-malignant lesions[15]. In contrast, the low-risk strains HPV 6 and 11 are not oncogenic but are thought to cause about 90% of genital warts. The existence of a limited number of carcinogenic strains has been of central importance in development of a vaccine as protection against cervical cancer. There are two vaccines currently available; Cervarix™ (GlaxoSmithKline Biologicals) is bivalent, protecting against the high-risk HPV 16 and 18 strains, whereas Gardasil™ (Sanofi Pasteur MSD) is quadrivalent and also protects against the genital wart strains HPV 6 and 11[16]. Most commentators concur that HPV 6 and 11 are included in the quadrivalent vaccine in the hope that this will encourage parents of boys to take up the vaccine. Although the impact on male health might be slight, by reducing the pool of infectious males, it is likely that this would help to protect unvaccinated women. This is further discussed in 'Prevention' section.

Biology

All HPV share certain characteristics; they have a small circular single-stranded DNA genome which codes for just eight proteins. The primary oncogenes are E6 and E7 and a key event in carcinogenesis is an increase in the levels of the oncoproteins for which they code. In cells of the cervical epithelium the genome is found episomally; in early stages of infection it occurs as a circular single strand of DNA; in malignant cervical lesions it is found integrated into host cell DNA[17].

Squamous epithelium[18,19]

Papillomaviruses are highly species-specific and only infect 'stratified epithelia of the skin, the anogenital tract and the oral cavity'[5]. It may therefore be helpful to review the features of stratified squamous epithelium, which is the type found in these locations.

There are several types of epithelium; those which are relevant for this discussion are squamous epithelium, which may be simple or stratified, and simple columnar epithelium which consists of a single layer of cells shaped like columns, and is found adjacent to squamous epithelium in the cervix.

Squamous epithelium has a surface of flattened scale-like cells – simple squamous epithelium has a single layer of these cells. In stratified squamous epithelium (SSE) there is a series of layers, with only the lowest layer in contact with the basement membrane. Successively more superficial layers are more flattened and scale-like. Stratified squamous epithelium occurs in anatomical sites where the surface may be subjected to mechanical abradement – put simply, where the top layer of cells may be worn away by friction. This type of epithelium may be keratinized – in which the topmost layer of cells is dead and is covered over with secreted keratin, which is a hard waterproof coating. Keratinized epithelium is found on the external surface of the body – the skin.

Internal surfaces lined with non-keratinized SSE include the oral cavity, the cervix, and the rectum – all sites in which HPV-associated cancer has been described. Even in non-keratinized SSE the epithelial cells are called keratinocytes; the lowest layers of these, which are in contact with the basement membrane, are referred to as basal cells or foot cells. The basal cells are the stem cell population; as they divide they produce a daughter cell which remains in contact with the basement membrane and a daughter cell which migrates to the external surface. As they migrate to the surface they become progressively more flattened. Normally, as they move upwards they undergo terminal differentiation – they lose the capacity to divide.

The life cycle of the papillomavirus is intimately linked to the process by which cells within the SSE progress to the surface and change their morphology. The virus exploits the keratinocyte differentiation pathway to evade immune recognition[20]. In the basal layer the virus is non-replicative and produces no virions, it expresses few genes (called the early genes) but these genes drive division of the basal cells. Only as cells near the surface and are ready to be shed does the virus trigger a replicative cycle leading to the shedding of virions – this is occurring in a region where there is little or no risk of triggering an immune response. This is only one of the mechanisms by which the virus evades an immune response but this, at least in part, explains the tropism for squamous epithelium.

HPV DNA is found in skin cancers both in immunocompetent individuals (30–50%) and immunosuppressed organ transplant recipients (~90%)[21]; the IARC review of HPV, however, concluded that there is only 'limited' evidence implicating HPV genus-beta types in the aetiology of skin cancer in the general population. Strikingly, the sites where HPV stands convicted as an unquestioned carcinogen all share an unusual anatomical feature – transformation zones. A transformation zone is a region where 'one kind of epithelium contacts and gradually replaces another by literally transforming itself through a process referred to as metaplasia'[22]. Transformation zones occur in the uterine cervix, in the anus and the tonsils; in each location HPV-associated cancers occur in the transformation zone, even though HPV DNA may be detectable in adjacent tissues[22]. Striking evidence is provided by a comparison of the incidence of penile cancer and of cervical cancer – although males have a higher rate of genital warts, incidence of penile cancer is an order of magnitude lower than that of cervical cancer. This is true even in countries where cervical cancer screening has been in place for 40 years or more. There are two plausible factors which may explain this. Firstly, the cervix, unlike the penis, has a large transformation zone[23] and secondly, clearance of HPV infection in men is rapid, especially for high-risk strains[24].

The transformation zone of the cervix is very well delineated; the outer region of the cervix is contiguous with the vaginal epithelium and is covered with non-keratinized SSE, the inner region is contiguous with the uterine lining and is covered with simple columnar epithelium[25]. The region of change from one to the other is known as the squamocolumnar junction and is the zone in which most cancers occur; it is this region which is sampled by a successful 'smear test'[26]. In young women the junctional region is low on the ectocervix but it 'migrates' upwards into the cervical canal with increasing age; this is significant because high-risk HPV species preferentially colonize the junctional region[27].

Epidemiology/transmission

HPV strains are exquisitely adapted to their host organism and to their preferred anatomical site within that organism – different strains are typically found on the mucosa and within the skin[14]. Transmission is by intimate skin–skin, skin–mucosa or mucosa–mucosa contact; in the case of anogenital infection, sexual transmission is overwhelmingly the most common route[28]. It has been suggested in the past that condoms are ineffective in preventing transmission of HPV[29]; although they are less effective than with some other STIs, consistent condom use markedly reduces the risk of transmission[30–33].

Another factor which reduces transmission is male circumcision, the incidence of penile lesions is lower in circumcised males[34], as is the incidence of cervical cancer in their female partners[35,36]. It has been suggested that the higher risk of penile cancer in uncircumcised males is related to a higher incidence of phimosis in this group; when the analysis only included men who did not report a history of phimosis the protective effect was lost[37,38]; timing of circumcision is important, only being protective if done during the neonatal period[39]. In a US study the protective effect against cervical cancer was seen only for partners of men with high risk behaviour, defined as intercourse before 17, six or more sexual partners or history of contact with prostitutes[40]; where both male and female partners were at low risk of infection there was no protective effect of circumcision.

Anogenital HPV infection is strongly correlated with sexual activity but need not involve penetrative sex, as evidenced by infections in women who have sex with women[41,42]. It has been observed in situations where it is clear that non-sexual transmission is the only plausible route, including cases in children where careful review concluded that child sexual abuse was highly unlikely[43].

It has long been held that nuns do not get cervical cancer and that it is only seen in sexually active women – this was based on Rigoni-Stern's report in the mid-nineteenth century[44], but this has been robustly challenged by Griffiths, in a paper challenging the DoH policy (in 1990) of not screening *'nuns, virgins and spinsters'*[45]. Griffiths cited a series of studies which showed that the rate of cervical cancer in nuns is not markedly less than in the general population of single women.

It is clear that only a very low percentage of HPV-infected women go on to develop cervical lesions; in the overwhelming majority of cases the infection is cleared, probably by the a cell-mediated immune response[46]. Follow up of detected infections indicates that more than 90% clear up within 2 years[22]. In a minority of women the virus will establish a long-term, asymptomatic latent infection; if infection with a high-risk strain persists for more than a year, there is an increased risk of cervical cancer[47]. A recent study, still to be confirmed, suggests that inherited variations of a specific innate immune gene (IRF3) are associated with increased risk of persistence of HPV infection[48]; inherited variations in another gene (FANCA) were reported, in the same study, to be associated with variation in the risk of progression to cervical cancer. Although cervical cancer represents a very small tip of a very large pyramid, the large number of women at risk means that cervical cancer is *'the third most common cancer in women worldwide, with an estimated incidence of about 470 000 cases in 2000, and the second most common in developing countries, where it accounts for about 15% of all cancers in women'*[49,50].

The incidence of infection with skin-tropic HPV strains is probably even higher and is independent of sexual behaviour; it has been suggested that 'probably everybody is infected over long periods, if not throughout life, with these viruses'[51]. Fortunately, these strains are usually non-carcinogenic in immunocompetent individuals, although compromised immunity is associated with an excess of skin cancer, probably HPV-initiated[52]. Demonstration of HPV DNA in squamous skin cancers from immunocompetent individuals suggests that immunocompromise may not be a prerequisite for progression to cancer[53].

Associated malignancies

Globally, by far the most important HPV-associated cancer is cancer of the uterine cervix. Cervical cancer was the first cancer to be shown to be invariably associated with a specific infectious agent – 99.7% of tumours can be shown to be HPV positive[54], the remaining 0.3% are presumed to be false-negatives due to technical failures. Anal cancers and a subset of head and neck cancers are causally linked with high-risk HPV infection.

Screening for, and ablation of, cervical pre-malignant lesions has dramatically reduced the incidence of cervical cancer in the developed world – 80% of cervical cancer deaths occur in the developing world[55]. The developed world is, in contrast, seeing a steady increase in incidence of anal[56] and of HPV-linked head and neck cancer[57], the latter possibly linked with changing sexual behaviour[58]. The increase in head and neck cancer is not an artefact of improved diagnosis as there is no concomitant increase in the rate of non-HPV-associated cancer in this area.

Cervical cancer

As stated, cervical cancer is one of the commonest cancers globally, with a particularly high incidence in the developing world. As recently as the 1930s it was the leading cause of cancer death for women in the US[59]; this situation was transformed by the introduction of screening programmes to detect and treat premalignant lesions (described in detail in 'Prevention' section).

The pathways leading from initial infection with HPV high-risk strains to invasive cervical cancer are now largely outlined[60], but many questions remain to be answered. *'An estimated 30–60% of sexually active men and women are infected with genital HPV, largely asymptomatically. Progression from clinically detectable infection to invasive cervical carcinoma occurs in less than 1% of women'*[20]. The sine qua non is infection with HPV; the epidemiological evidence suggests that this is extremely common but that around 90% of all infections resolve spontaneously within 2 years – an obvious question is why some infections persist. Even Harald zur Hausen, who shared the 2008 Nobel Prize for 'his discovery of human papilloma viruses causing cervical cancer', has stated that *'Although more than 95% of cervical cancer biopsies contain high risk HPV genomes, this figure does not necessarily imply that all of these tumors are caused by these infections. Long-term follow-up studies of vaccinated women, particularly after achieving a broad protection against the majority of high risk HPV types, will provide a better basis for more accurate estimates'*[61]. Notwithstanding this note of caution, cervical carcinomas have been described as '*... unfortunate complications of longstanding infections with high-risk types of human papillomavirus (hrHPV)'*[62].

The natural history of cervical cancer involves a series of stages of increasing malignant potential leading to invasive cervical cancer[15]. There are two main schemes currently used to describe these stages[63].

Standard approach[64,65]

- Normal
- Inflammatory
- Cervical intraepithelial neoplasia
  - Stage one
  - Stage two
  - Stage three
- Invasive cervical cancer

Bethesda classification[66]

- Normal
- Inflammatory

■ Atypical squamous cells
  o Of undetermined significance (ASC-US)
  o Cannot exclude high-grade (ASC-H)
■ Squamous intraepithelial lesions
  o Low grade (LGSIL)
  o High grade (HGSIL)
■ Squamous cell carcinoma (SCC)

In the Bethesda classification LGSIL equates to CIN1, with CIN2 and 3 subsumed into HGSIL. LGSIL/CIN1 may be caused by low-risk HPV strains and often resolve spontaneously; they are not an indication for surgery. HGSIL/CIN3 each incorporates carcinoma *in situ*, defined by WHO as '*a lesion in which all or most of the epithelium shows the cellular features of carcinoma*'[67]; Koss defines it as '*an intraepithelial lesion histologically resembling invasive cervical cancer*'[68]. Koss's definition has the merit of explicitly indicating the differentiating feature – a lack of invasion of neighbouring tissues.

Establishment of persistent infection with a high-risk strain is associated with a high probability of eventual malignancy[47], but this occurs after a long period of latency. It is not clear whether a specific trigger(s) is involved but an elegant study using data from a Swedish population register indicated a genetic component[69,70]. Epidemiological evidence indicates that over 90% of carcinoma *in situ* (early stage cervical cancer) is registered in women under 45 with a peak in the 25–29 age group – this reflects the estimated latency following establishment of persistent infection.

Invasive cervical cancer is, in contrast more nearly equal in rates above the age of 25 years but with two striking peaks, which represent those cohorts of women who were born at the end of the nineteenth century and around 1920 and would have become sexually active around the time of World War I and World War II[71]. The probability of persistent infection with high-risk strains is greater in women who have sex with men with high numbers of sexual partners[72]; in many societies women have little or no control over the sexual behaviour of their partners, which in turn gives them no direct control over this risk factor.

Cofactors
A number of cofactors have been reported[73,74];

■ Five or more years oral contraceptive use
■ Cigarette smoking
■ More than five full-term pregnancies
■ Co-infection with other STIs
  o *Chlamydia trachomatis*
  o Herpes simplex virus type 2 (HSV-2).
■ Dietary factors
■ Multiple sexual partners, early first intercourse[75]
■ High-risk male partner[36], especially if he is uncircumcised
■ Poverty[76]

Cigarette smoking has been difficult to establish as a cofactor rather than a confounder because smoking is strongly associated with low socio-economic status, which is linked in turn with early first sexual activity and multiple partners[77]. A meta-analysis of 23 studies by the International Collaboration of Epidemiological Studies of Cervical Cancer concluded smoking to be a risk factor for squamous cell cancer of the cervix[78].

Women exposed to the human immunodeficiency virus (HIV) are at high risk for having persistent high-risk HPV infection and for progression to invasive cervical cancer, the excess risk appears to persist in women receiving HAART, even though HAART reduces the risk of Kaposi sarcoma and of non-Hodgkin lymphoma[79]. Although the evidence for an increased risk appears robust[80,81], the HAART results suggest that there may be a more complex mechanism than simple immunosuppression. It is probable that, once persistent high-risk HPV infection has been established, elimination of HIV infection is irrelevant; this would be analogous to the behaviour of gastric MALToma which, in early stages, is *Helicobacter pylori* dependent but, in later stages, will progress even if the bacterial infection is eradicated.

Prevention

Historically, prevention has been secondary, as there was no way to protect sexually active women from acquiring the infection. Screening programmes using the Papanicolaou smear detected pre-malignant lesions and allowed intervention to prevent malignant transformation.

Cervical cancer is an illness ideally suited to prevention by screening:

- The natural history is well understood
- There is a reliable and sensitive screening test available
- There is a long period between appearance of initial lesions and development of invasive cancer
- Treatment of pre-malignant lesions is curative

It should be noted that none of these criteria depended on identification of the causative agent; screening was underway long before the link between cervical cancer and HPV had been demonstrated. The crucial prerequisite for an effective screening programme was the development, by George Papanicolaou, of the now ubiquitous 'Pap smear'. He published a paper in 1928 describing his observations of uterine cancer cells in vaginal fluids[82]; this was followed in 1941 by the first description of the diagnostic method which became central to mass-screening programmes[83].

There is a wide global variation in the prevalence of HPV infection and in the proportions of high-risk infections[84]. There is a strong correlation between HPV prevalence and cervical cancer incidence; in the developed world this may be obscured by the efficacy of screening programmes in preventing invasive cancer. Peto *et al.*[85] have said that '*Cervical screening has prevented an epidemic that would have killed about one in 65 of all British women born since 1950 and culminated in about 6000 deaths per year in this country'* and *'about 100 000 (one in 80) of the 8 million British women born between 1951 and 1970 will be saved from premature death by the cervical screening programme at a cost per life saved of about £36 000'*. It is not universally accepted that screening programmes are the explanation for declining cervical cancer rates – some have challenged whether they have any value; a recent review discusses both sides of the debate[86]. There is very wide international variation in the coverage and effectiveness of screening programmes[87].

Emphasis is now moving towards primary prevention by vaccination against high-risk strains of HPV. In the UK the chosen vaccine (Cervarix) is effective against HPV 16 and 18, which together are thought to account for about 70% of invasive cancer and about 50% of pre-malignant lesions. In the US, Gardasil has been preferred, which also protects against HPV 6 and 11, which are considered low-risk for cervical cancer but account for about 90% of genital warts. Both vaccines are based on self-assembling mixtures of L1 virus proteins which form virus-like-particles (VLPs)[88]. The L1 protein is the principal epitope which determines vaccine specificity. Because neither of the vaccines uses complete viruses, live or inactivated, they are safe for use in potentially immunosuppressed subjects.

Even the quadrivalent vaccine is only predicted to prevent about 70% of potentially oncogenic infections[89], on this basis it has been stressed that screening for pre-malignant lesions will continue to be necessary indefinitely[26]. An additional reason for caution is the lack of reliable data on how long protection will last[90]. A 2009 paper on a prospective study on close to 18 000 women reported that the quadrivalent vaccine also reduced the risk of pre-malignant lesions associated with non-vaccine types responsible for about 20% of cervical cancer. An important caveat was that, *'clinical benefit of cross-protection is not expected to be fully additive to the efficacy already observed against HPV-6/11/16/18-related disease, because women may have >1 CIN lesion, each associated with a different HPV type'*[91]. This report may not be relevant to the UK situation, as the UK government has decided that the NHS will supply the bivalent vaccine, which may offer less, or no, cross protection. A second generation of HPV vaccines is under development; the goal of researchers is to develop *'cheap, thermostable vaccines that can be delivered by noninjectable methods that provide long-term (decades) protection at mucosal surfaces to most, if not all, oncogenic HPV types that is as good as the current VLP vaccines'*[92].

HPV vaccination may prove of greatest value in populations where male promiscuity is commonplace and where women have little or no ability to control partner behaviour. Although this is very commonly the case in the developing world, it is also true of disadvantaged socio-economic groups in developed countries. There is evidence that male circumcision reduces the level of penile HPV infection and the risk of cervical cancer in female partners[40].

Routine Pap screening among younger women received a boost in early 2009; this followed the death of reality TV star Jade Goody from metastatic cervical cancer, and was attributed to the very extensive publicity surrounding her illness[93]. It is controversial whether the potential health benefits of screening younger women outweighs the adverse effects of surgical extirpation of lesions which are very likely to spontaneously resolve. Many women in this age group will have LGSL/ CIN1 lesions, which rarely progress to invasive cancer. The 2008 review of the cervical screening programme explains the rationale for starting screening at 25 years[94]; this policy is under review at the time of writing – further information can be found at http://www.cancerscreening.nhs.uk/cervical/index.html. A 2006 paper compared the UK policy of screening women 3 yearly from 20 to 64 years with the Australian policy of screening 2 yearly from 18 to 69 years and found them to be of *'broadly similar effectiveness'*[87]. A mathematical model published in 2010[95] suggested that diminished screening due to vaccination is unlikely to lead to increased cases, that screening would continue to be necessary, but that it may be possible to increase intervals for screening.

Other genital cancers

Cancers of the vagina, vulva and penis have all been associated with HPV infection, particularly with the HPV 16 high-risk strain[5].

Penis

Cancer of the penis is at least an order of magnitude less common than cancer of the cervix and this remains true even in populations where the incidence of cervical cancer has been lowered by universal screening programmes[96]. There is a marked geographical correlation between incidence of cervical cancer and that of penile cancer[96], and also significant concordance of these cancers between spouses[97].

The estimates of the contribution of HPV to penile cancer vary quite widely[97], possibly because the association is most marked in the more aggressive SCC form of the cancer[98], some studies have included high numbers of SCC and may, therefore, have overestimated the contribution of HPV[99]. Reviews tend to concur on an estimate of about half of all penile cancers being HPV-associated[96,100].

There are three forms of penile carcinoma *in situ*, which correspond to cervical intraepithelial neoplasia; these are Bowen's disease, erythroplasia of Queyrat and Bowenoid papulosis. Erythroplasia of Queyrat is the term traditionally applied to Bowen's disease affecting the glans of the penis[101]. Bowen's disease and erythroplasia of Queyrat may progress to invasive SCC; Bowenoid papulosis is typically a benign lesion encountered in young sexually active individuals[101-103]. Despite the benign reputation of Bowenoid papulosis there are (rare) reports of malignant progression and it has been recommended that lesions should be excised to avoid this outcome[104]. Both pre-malignant lesions and invasive SCC are more frequently associated with HPV 16 than with other HPV types[105-107].

Cofactors

Etiological factors associated with penile cancer are phimosis, chronic inflammatory conditions, especially lichen sclerosus, smoking, ultraviolet irradiation, history of warts, or condylomas and lack of circumcision[101]. As indicated, only about half of penile cancers are HPV-associated; this makes it difficult to determine to what extent other risk factors are primary causes or cofactors with HPV.

Prevention

Primary prevention is based upon prevention of infection with HPV high-risk strains. Early circumcision has been reported to reduce the incidence of HPV infection and of penile neoplasms in men[108], although some studies report that this is only true when the operation is carried out in infancy[37]. A recent editorial in *Journal of Infectious Diseases* discusses the sometimes conflicting evidence on circumcision[109]. In some instances cultural or logistical problems may complicate this approach[110].

Anal cancer[111]

Anal cancer is uncommon, but the incidence has been reported to be rising over the last half-century[56,112–115]. Although incidence in the general population is low, the incidence in men who have sex with men (MSM) is higher than that for cervical cancer in the general population of women[112]. An Australian review reported that in MSM overall the rate of anal cancer is at least 20 times higher than in the general population but concluded that there was no evidence to support a general screening programme in MSM for anal cancer[116]. A US review recommended that high risk populations, defined as '*all HIV-positive women and men, MSM, women with a history of vulvar or cervical cancer and organ transplant recipients*'[100], should be routinely screened to permit early detection of anal cancer.

The association between anal cancer and HPV infection is strong and consistent. HPV 16 is the most common HPV type associated with anal cancer. In cervical cancer both HPV 16 and HPV 18 are deemed by IARC as definitely carcinogenic in human; in anal cancer HPV 16 is classed as a definite carcinogen but HPV 18 is only classed as possibly carcinogenic[5]. It is estimated that over 80% of all cases of anal cancer are associated with HPV infection[117].

Cofactors

Known risk factors include, anoreceptive intercourse, cigarette smoking and immunosuppression[111]. The contribution of HIV infection is unclear, although anal cancer is more common in HIV positive men; there is a strong correlation between HPV positivity and HIV positivity[118]. Anal HPV positivity has been reported in about a quarter of heterosexual men[119], with a third of these infections being high-risk strains; it may be that the high disparity between anal cancer rates in MSM and other men is at least partly due to differences in incidence of cofactors.

Prevention

Whether to routinely screen for anal cancer among MSM is a controversial issue; as is the question of what method might be appropriate[120–125]. A UK study[126] concluded, based on 2008 incidence and available methods that it would cost between

£20 996 and £39 405 per quality adjusted life year (QALY) gained; this should be compared against the NICE threshold of £30 000 per QALY applied when assessing new cancer drugs. The study, perhaps unsurprisingly, concluded that further studies and better data were needed, and that these might establish cost effectiveness of screening in high-risk groups.

Head and neck cancer[127,128]

'Head and neck cancer is a broad term that encompasses epithelial malignancies that arise in the paranasal sinuses, nasal cavity, oral cavity, pharynx, and larynx'[127]. More than 90% of these are squamous cell cancers (HNSCC), with the major known risk factors being smoking and alcohol[129]. About a quarter of HNSCC appears to be caused by HPV infection, mainly the high risk strains HPV 16 and to a lesser extent HPV 18[127,128]. There are significant differences in the anatomical locations of HPV positive and negative HNSCC; the HPV positive cancers are found mainly in the areas of the tonsils and the base of the tongue[130], regions where there are transformation zones.

Patients with HPV high-risk positive HNSCC have a better prognosis than those with HPV negative disease, with lower rates of relapse and of second tumours[131,132].

Cofactors

Unlike HPV negative HNSCC, HPV positive cases are not associated with smoking or alcohol, indeed negative correlations have been reported[133,134]; patients in these studies were also younger, which may in part explain better clinical outcomes.

Prevention

The primary pathway for transmission of high-risk HPV strains causing HNSCC is thought to be oral sex[135-139]. Some studies have indicated that adolescents are more inclined to engage in oral than vaginal sex, probably in response to health education campaigns on avoiding pregnancy and on HIV risks. 'Given that adolescents perceive oral sex as less risky, more prevalent, and more acceptable than vaginal sex, it stands to reason that adolescents are more likely to engage in oral sex'[140]. A survey of adolescents reported perceptions of the consequences of oral versus vaginal sex concluded, 'adolescents who engaged only in oral sex were less likely to report experiencing a pregnancy or sexually transmitted infection, feeling guilty or used, having their relationship become worse, and getting into trouble with their parents as a result of sex. Adolescents who engaged only in oral sex were also less likely to report experiencing pleasure, feeling good about themselves, and having their relationship become better as a result of sex'[141]. It is probable that education campaigns will have limited impact on adolescent behaviour, and these findings may prove persuasive for the extension of HPV vaccination to include young males. In a US study of men's attitudes towards receiving the HPV vaccine, one-third of men provided with information were willing to be vaccinated and 40% of this group cited protection against

HNSCC, anal or penile cancer as their reason[142]. A study of variables associated with male acceptance of HPV vaccination concluded, *'the availability of clinical research findings and a focused lay educational program should facilitate even wider HPV vaccine acceptance by men'*[143].

Summary

▪ Papillomaviruses have co-evolved with their host species and are capable of establishing and maintaining long-term asymptomatic infections
▪ There are more than 100 subtypes distinguished on the basis of DNA sequence, and over 40 strains are known to infect the human anogenital tract
▪ A high rate of infection with HPV is found in all geographical areas
   o A minority of these are classed as IARC Group 1 – definite carcinogenic in humans
   o HPV 16, 18, 31, 33, 35, 39, 45, 51, 52, 56, 58, 59, 66, HPV genus-beta types 5 and 8
▪ Rates of cervical cancer have been reduced in the developed world by programmes which screen for, and treat, pre-malignant lesions
   o The introduction of HPV vaccine covering the most ubiquitous carcinogenic strains is expected to further reduce the incidence of HPV-related cancer in developed nations
▪ In the developing world, HPV-related cervical cancer is a leading cause of female cancer mortality
▪ In HPV infection is associated with other ano-genital cancers and with a sub-set of head and neck cancer

In the developing world HPV-associated cervical cancer is a leading cause of female cancer mortality. Screening programmes for cervical cancer have reduced mortality, but not morbidity in developed world populations. Recently introduced vaccines against high risk strains of HPV, which are responsible for about 70% of cervical cancer, are expected to significantly reduce infection rates and hence morbidity and mortality. In the UK the government has chosen a bivalent vaccine, active against HPV 16 and 18; the US government has chosen a quadric-valent vaccine which is also effective against strains 6 and 11, which are low risk for cervical cancer but cause genital warts. The US policy is based, at least in part, on the expectation that protection against genital warts will encourage young males to seek vaccination, thus enhancing further protection against cervical cancer in their female partners.

References

1. Hampl, M. (2007) Prevention of human papilloma virus-induced preneoplasia and cancer by prophylactic HPV vaccines. *Minerva Medica*, **98**, 121–130.
2. Brisson, M., Van de, V, De Wals, P. & Boily, M.C. (2007) Estimating the number needed to vaccinate to prevent diseases and death related to human papillomavirus infection. *Canadian Medical Association Journal*, **177**, 464–468.

3. IARC Working Group on the Evaluation of Cancer Prevention Strategies (2004) Cervix cancer screening. IARC Press, Lyon.

4. Economist Intelligence Unit (2009) *Breakaway: The Global Burden of Cancer.* Economic Intelligence Unit, London.

5. IARC Working Group on the Evaluation of Carcinogenic Risks to Humans (2005) *Human Papillomaviruses*, Vol. 90. Lyon, France.

6. Alos, L., Moyano, S., Nadal, A., *et al.* (2009) Human papillomaviruses are identified in a subgroup of sinonasal squamous cell carcinomas with favorable outcome. *Cancer*, **115**, 2701–2709.

7. Baumann, J.L., Cohen, S., Evjen, A.N., *et al.* (2009) Human papillomavirus in early laryngeal carcinoma. *Laryngoscope*, **119**, 1531–1537.

8. Dreilich, M., Bergqvist, M., Moberg, M., *et al.* (2006) High-risk human papilloma virus (HPV) and survival in patients with esophageal carcinoma: A pilot study. *BMC Cancer*, **6**, 94.

9. Frazer, I.H. (2009) Interaction of human papillomaviruses with the host immune system: A well evolved relationship. *Virology*, **384**, 410–414.

10. Galloway, D.A. (2009) Human papillomaviruses: A growing field. *Genes & Development*, **23**, 138–142.

11. Howley, P.M. & Livingston, D.M. (2009) Small DNA tumor viruses: Large contributors to biomedical sciences. *Virology*, **384**, 256–259.

12. Bernard, H.U. (2005) The clinical importance of the nomenclature, evolution and taxonomy of human papillomaviruses. *Journal of Clinical Virology*, **32S**, S1–S6.

13. Andrewes, C. (1964) Tumour-viruses and virus-tumours. *BMJ*, **1**, 653–658.

14. de Villiers, E.M., Fauquet, C., Broker, T.R., Bernard, H.U. & zur Hausen, H. (2004) Classification of papillomaviruses. *Virology*, **324**, 17–27.

15. Schiffman, M., Castle, P.E., Jeronimo, J., Rodriguez, A.C. & Wacholder, S. (2007) Human papillomavirus and cervical cancer. *Lancet*, **370**, 890–907.

16. Scientific Panel on the guidance for the introduction of HPV vaccines in EU countries (2008) *Guidance for the Introduction of HPV Vaccines in EU Countries.* European Centre for Disease Prevention and Control, Stockholun.

17. Hudelist, G., Manavi, M., Pischinger, K.I., *et al.* (2004) Physical state and expression of HPV DNA in benign and dysplastic cervical tissue: Different levels of viral integration are correlated with lesion grade. *Gynecologic Oncology*, **2**, 873–880.

18. Faller, A., Schünke, M. & Schünke, G. (2004) Tissues. In: *The Human Body: An Introduction to Structure and Function* (eds A. Faller, M. Schünke & G. Schünke), pp. 67–112. Thieme, Stuttgart.

19. Wheater, P.R., Burkitt, H.G. & Daniels, V.G. (1987) Epithelial tissues. In: *Functional Histology: A Text and Colour Atlas* (eds P.R. Wheater, H.G. Burkitt & V.G. Daniels), pp. 64–78. Churchill Livingstone, Edinburgh.

20. Tindle, R.W. (2002) Immune evasion in human papillomavirus-associated cervical cancer. *Nature Reviews Cancer*, **2**, 59–65.

21. Munoz, N., Castellsague, X., de Gonzalez, A.B. & Gissmann, L. (2006) Chapter 1: HPV in the etiology of human cancer. *Vaccine*, **24** (Suppl. 3), S1–S10.

22. Moscicki, A.B., Schiffman, M., Kjaer, S. & Villa, L.L. (2006) Chapter 5: Updating the natural history of HPV and anogenital cancer. *Vaccine*, **24** (Suppl. 3), S42–S51.

23. Partridge, J.M. & Koutsky, L.A. (2006) Genital human papillomavirus infection in men. *Lancet Infectious Diseases*, **6**, 21–31.

24. Giuliano, A.R., Lu, B., Nielson, C.M., *et al.* (2008) Age-specific prevalence, incidence, and duration of human papillomavirus infections in a cohort of 290 US men. *Journal of Infectious Diseases*, **198**, 827–835.

25. Wheater, P.R., Burkitt, H.G. & Daniels, V.G. (1987) Female reproductive system. In: *Functional Histology: A Text and Colour Atlas* (eds P.R. Wheater, H.G. Burkitt & V.G. Daniels), pp. 289–307. Churchill Livingstone, Edinburgh.

26. Warren, J.B., Gullett, H. & King, V.J. (2009) Cervical cancer screening and updated pap guidelines. *Primary Care*, **36**, 131–149, ix.

27. Castle, P.E., Jeronimo, J., Schiffman, M., *et al.* (2006) Age-related changes of the cervix influence human papillomavirus type distribution. *Cancer Research*, **66**, 1218–1224.

28. Bosch, F.X., Qiao, Y.L. & Castellsague, X. (2006) The epidemiology of human papillomavirus infection and its association with cervical cancer. *International Journal of Gynecology and Obstetrics*, **94**, S8–S21.

29. Gerberding, J.L. (2004) *Prevention of Genital Human Papillomavirus Infection – A Report to Congress*. Center for Disease Control and Prevention, Atlanta, GA.

30. Epstein, R.J. (2005) Primary prevention of human papillomavirus-dependent neoplasia: No condom, no sex. *European Journal of Cancer*, **41**, 2595–2600.

31. Moscicki, A.B. (2005) Impact of HPV infection in adolescent populations. *Journal of Adolescent Health*, **37**, S3–S9.

32. Weaver, B.A. (2006) Epidemiology and natural history of genital human papillomavirus infection. *Journal of the American Osteopathic Association*, **106**, S2–S8.

33. Winer, R., Hughes, J.P., Feng, Q., *et al.* (2006) Consistent condom use from time of first vaginal intercourse and the risk of genital human papillomavirus infection in young women. *New England Journal of Medicine*, **354**, 2645–2654.

34. MacLean, R. (2005) Odds of penile HPV are reduced for circumcised men and condom users. *International Family Planning Perspectives*, **31**, 42.

35. Chou, P. (1991) Review on risk factors of cervical cancer. *Zhonghua Yi Xue Za Zhi (Taipei)*, **48**, 81–88.

36. Kjaer, S.K., de Villiers, E.M., Dahl, C., *et al.* (1991) Case-control study of risk factors for cervical neoplasia in Denmark. I: Role of the "male factor" in women with one lifetime sexual partner. *International Journal of Cancer*, **48**, 39–44.

37. Daling, J.R., Madeleine, M.M., Johnson, L.G., *et al.* (2005) Penile cancer: Importance of circumcision, human papillomavirus and smoking in in situ and invasive disease. *International Journal of Cancer*, **116**, 606–616.

38. Tsen, H.F., Morgenstern, H., Mack, T. & Peters, R.K. (2001) Risk factors for penile cancer: Results of a population-based case-control study in Los Angeles County (United States). *Cancer Causes & Control*, **12**, 267–277.

39. Maden, C., Sherman, K.J., Beckmann, A.M., *et al.* (1993) History of circumcision, medical conditions, and sexual activity and risk of penile cancer. *Journal of the National Cancer Institute*, **85**, 19–24.

40. Castellsague, X., Bosch, F.X., Munoz, N., *et al.* (2002) Male circumcision, penile papillomavirus infection and cervical cancer in female partners. *The New England Journal of Medicine*, **346**, 1105–1112.

41. Marrazzo, J.M., Stine, K. & Koutsky, L.A. (2000) Genital human papillomavirus in women who have sex with women: A review. *American Journal of Obstetrics & Gynecology*, **183**, 770–774.

42. Marrazzo, J.M., Koutsky, L.A., Kiviat, N.B., Kuypers, J.M. & Stine, K. (2001) Papanicolaou test screening and prevalence of genital human papillomavirus among women who have sex with women. *American Journal of Public Health*, **91**, 947–952.

43. Sinclair, K.A., Woods, C.R., Kirse, D.J. & Sinal, S.H. (2005) Anogenital and respiratory tract human papillomavirus infections among children: Age, gender, and potential transmission through sexual abuse. *Pediatrics*, **116**, 815–825.

44. Rigoni-Stern & Transl. by de Stavola, B. (1987) Statistical facts about cancers on which Dr Rigoni-Stern based his contribution to the surgeon's subgroup of the IV congress of the Italian scientists on 23rd September 1842. Originally published in *Giornale par servire al Progressi della Patologia e della Terapeutica*, Ser 2, Vol 2, pp 507–517 (1842). *Statistics in Medicine*, **6**, 881–884.

45. Griffiths, M. (1991) 'Nuns, virgins and spinsters'. Rigoni-Stern and cervical cancer revisited. *BJOG*, **98**, 797–802.

46. Stanley, M. (2008) Immunobiology of HPV and HPV vaccines. *Gynecologic Oncology*, **109**, S15–S21.

47. Ho, G.Y., Burk, R.D., Klein, S., *et al.* (1995) Persistent genital human papillomavirus infection as a risk factor for persistent cervical dysplasia. *Journal of the National Cancer Institute*, **87**, 1365–1371.

48. Wang, S.S., Bratti, M.C., Rodriguez, A.C., *et al.* (2009) Common variants in immune and DNA repair genes and risk for human papillomavirus persistence and progression to cervical cancer. *Journal of Infectious Diseases*, **199**, 20–30.

49. Drain, P.K., Holmes, K.K., Hughes, J.P. & Koutsky, L.A. (2002) Determinants of cervical cancer rates in developing countries. *International Journal of Cancer*, **100**, 199–205.

50. Parkin, D.M. (2006) The global health burden of infection-associated cancers in the year 2002. *International Journal of Cancer*, **118**, 3030–3044.

51. Bosch, F.X., Rohan, T., Schneider, A., *et al.* (2001) Papillomavirus research update: Highlights of the Barcelona HPV 2000 international papillomavirus conference. *Journal of Clinical Pathology*, **54**, 163–175.

52. Boukamp, P. (2005) Non-melanoma skin cancer: What drives tumor development and progression? *Carcinogenesis*, **26**, 1657–1667.

53. Purdie, K.J., Surentheran, T., Sterling, J.C., *et al.* (2005) Human papillomavirus gene expression in cutaneous squamous cell carcinomas from immunosuppressed and immunocompetent individuals. *Journal of Investigative Dermatology*, **125**, 98–107.

54. Walboomers, J.M., Jacobs, M.V., Manos, M.M., *et al.* (1999) Human papillomavirus is a necessary cause of invasive cervical cancer worldwide. *Journal of Pathology*, **189**, 12–19.

55. WHO (2002) *Cervical Cancer Screening in Developing Countries: Report of a WHO Consultation*. World Health Organization, Geneva.

56. Robinson, D., Coupland, V. & Moller, H. (2009) An analysis of temporal and generational trends in the incidence of anal and other HPV-related cancers in Southeast England. *British Journal of Cancer*, **100**, 527–531.

57. Haddad, R.I. & Shin, D.M. (2008) Recent advances in head and neck cancer. *New England Journal of Medicine*, **359**, 1143–1154.

58. Mosher, W.D., Chandra, A. & Jones, J. (2005) Sexual behavior and selected health measures: Men and women 15–44 years of age, United States, 2002. *Advance Data*, **15**, 1–55.

59. American College of Obstetricians and Gynecologists (2003) ACOG practice bulletin: Clinical management guidelines for obstetrician-gynecologists. Number 45, August 2003. Cervical cytology screening (replaces committee opinion 152, March 1995). *Obstetrics & Gynecology*, **102**, 417–427.

60. zur Hausen, H. (2002) Papillomaviruses and cancer: From basic studies to clinical application. *Nature Reviews Cancer*, **2**, 342–350.

61. zur Hausen H. (2009) Papillomaviruses in the causation of human cancers – A brief historical account. *Virology*, **384**, 260–265.

62. Bulk, S., Berkhof, J., Bulkmans, N.W., *et al.* (2006) Preferential risk of HPV16 for squamous cell carcinoma and of HPV18 for adenocarcinoma of the cervix compared to women with normal cytology in The Netherlands. *British Journal of Cancer*, **94**, 171–175.

63. Smith, J.R. & Barron, B.A. (1998) Cervical cancer. In: *Fast Facts: Gynaecological Oncology*, pp. 6–22. Oxford Health Press Ltd, Oxford.

64. Richart, R.M. (1973) Cervical intraepithelial neoplasia. *Pathology Annual*, **8**, 301–328.

65. Buckley, C.H., Butler, E.B. & Fox, H. (1982) Cervical intraepithelial neoplasia. *Journal of Clinical Pathology*, **35**, 1–13.

66. Solomon, D., Davey, D., Kurman, R., *et al.* (2002) The 2001 Bethesda system: Terminology for reporting results of cervical cytology. *JAMA*, **287**, 2114–2119.

67. Poulsen, H.E., Taylor, C.W. & Sobin, L.H. (1975) *Histological Typing of Female Genital Tract Tumours*. World Health Organisation, Geneva, pp. 55–57.

68. Koss, L.G. (1978) Dysplasia. A real concept or a misnomer? *Obstetrics & Gynecology*, **51**, 374–379.

69. Magnusson, P.K., Sparen, P. & Gyllensten, U.B. (1999) Genetic link to cervical tumours. *Nature*, **400**, 29–30.

70. Magnusson, P.K. & Gyllensten, U.B. (2000) Cervical cancer risk: Is there a genetic component? *Molecular Medicine Today*, **6**, 145–148.

71. Cancer Research UK (2003) *CancerStats – Cervical Cancer – UK*. Cancer Research UK, London.

72. Bosch, F.X. & Iftner, T. (2005) Epidemiology of human papillomavirus and cervical cancer. In: *The Aetiology of Cervical Cancer* (eds F.X. Bosch & T. Iftner), pp. 17–39. NHS Cancer Screening Programmes, Sheffield.

73. Bosch, F.X. & de Sanjose, S. (2007) The epidemiology of human papillomavirus infection and cervical cancer. *Disease Markers*, **23**, 213–227.

74. Trottier, H. & Franco, E.L. (2006) The epidemiology of genital human papillomavirus infection. *Vaccine*, **24** (Suppl. 1), S1–S15.

75. Murthy, N.S. & Mathew, A. (2000) Risk factors for pre-cancerous lesions of the cervix. *European Journal of Cancer Prevention*, **9**, 5–14.

76. Fletcher, H.M. & Hanchard, B. (2008) Poverty eradication and decreased human papilloma virus related cancer of the penis and vulva in Jamaica. *Journal of Obstetrics & Gynecology*, **28**, 333–335.

77. Syrjanen, K., Shabalova, I., Petrovichev, N., *et al.* (2007) Smoking is an independent risk factor for oncogenic human papillomavirus (HPV) infections but not for high-grade CIN. *European Journal of Epidemiology*, **22**, 723–735.

78. Appleby, P., Beral, V., Berrington de Gonzalez, A., *et al.* (2006) Carcinoma of the cervix and tobacco smoking: Collaborative reanalysis of individual data on 13,541 women with carcinoma of the cervix and 23,017 women without carcinoma of the cervix from 23 epidemiological studies. *International Journal of Cancer*, **118**, 1481–1495.

79. Clifford, G.M., Polesel, J., Rickenbach, M., *et al.* (2005) Cancer risk in the Swiss HIV cohort study: Associations with immunodeficiency, smoking, and highly active antiretroviral therapy. *Journal of National Cancer Institute*, **97**, 425–432.

80. Duerr, A., Paramsothy, P., Jamieson, D.J., *et al.* (2006) Effect of HIV infection on atypical squamous cells of undetermined significance. *Clinical Infectious Diseases*, **42**, 855–861.

81. Frega, A., Biamonti, A., Maranghi, L., *et al.* (2006) Follow-up of high-grade squamous intra-epithelial lesions (H-SILs) in human immunodeficiency virus (HIV)-positive and human papillomavirus (HPV)-positive women. Analysis of risk factors. *Anticancer Research*, **26**, 3167–3170.

82. Papanicolaou, G.N. (1928) New cancer diagnosis. In: *Proceedings of the Third Race Betterment Conference*, Race Betterment Foundation, Battle Creek, Michigan, pp. 528–534.

83. Papanicolaou, G.N. & Traut, H.F. (1941) The diagnostic value of vaginal smears in carcinoma of the uterus. *American Journal of Obstetrics & Gynecology*, **42**, 193–206.

84. Clifford, G.M., Gallus, S., Herrero, R., *et al.* (2005) Worldwide distribution of human papillomavirus types in cytologically normal women in the International Agency for Research on Cancer HPV prevalence surveys: A pooled analysis. *Lancet*, **366**, 991–998.

85. Peto, J., Gilham, C., Fletcher, O. & Matthews, F.E. (2004) The cervical cancer epidemic that screening has prevented in the UK. *Lancet*, **364**, 249–256.

86. Bryder, L. (2008) Debates about cervical screening: An historical overview. *Journal of Epidemiology & Community Health*, **62**, 284–287.

87. Gakidou, E., Nordhagen, S. & Obermeyer, Z. (2008) Coverage of cervical cancer screening in 57 countries: Low average levels and large inequalities. *PLoS Medicine*, **5**, e132.

88. Galloway, D.A. (2003) Papillomavirus vaccines in clinical trials. *Lancet Infectious Diseases*, **3**, 469–475.

89. Herzog, T.J., Huh, W.K., Downs, L.S., Smith, J.S. & Monk, B.J. (2008) Initial lessons learned in HPV vaccination. *Gynecologic Oncology*, **109**, S4–S11.

90. Schiller, J.T. & Lowy, D.R. (2006) Prospects for cervical cancer prevention by human papillomavirus vaccination. *Cancer Research*, **66**, 10229–10232.

91. Brown, D.R., Kjaer, S.K., Sigurdsson, K., *et al.* (2009) The impact of quadrivalent human papillomavirus (HPV; Types 6, 11, 16, and 18) L1 virus-like particle vaccine on infection and disease due to oncogenic nonvaccine HPV types in generally HPV-naive women aged 16–26 years. *Journal of Infectious Diseases*, **199**, 926–935.

92. Stanley, M. (2010) Prospects for new human papillomavirus vaccines. *Current Opinion in Infectious Diseases*, **23**, 70–75.

93. Cassidy, J. (2009) Jade, class, and cervical cancer. *BMJ*, **338**, b691.

94. Patnick, J. (2008) *NHS Cervical Screening Programme – Annual Review*. NHSCSP, Sheffield.

95. Li, M., Chapman, G., Galvani, A.P. & Li, M. (2010) Adherence to cervical screening in the era of human papillomavirus vaccination: How low is too low? *Lancet Infectious Diseases*, **10**, 133–137.

96. Parkin, D.M. & Bray, F. (2006) Chapter 2: The burden of HPV-related cancers. *Vaccine*, **24** (Suppl. 3), S11–S25.

97. Smith, P.G., Kinlen, L.J., White, G.C., Adelstein, A.M. & Fox, A.J. (1980) Mortality of wives of men dying with cancer of the penis. *British Journal of Cancer*, **41**, 422–428.

98. Gregoire, L., Cubilla, A.L., Reuter, V.E., Haas, G.P. & Lancaster, W.D. (1995) Preferential association of human papillomavirus with high-grade histologic variants of penile-invasive squamous cell carcinoma. *Journal of National Cancer Institute*, **87**, 1705–1709.

99. Chan, K.W., Lam, K.Y., Chan, A.C., Lau, P. & Srivastava, G. (1994) Prevalence of human papillomavirus types 16 and 18 in penile carcinoma: A study of 41 cases using PCR. *Journal of Clinical Pathology*, **47**, 823–826.

100. Palefsky, J.M. (2007) HPV infection in men. *Disease Markers*, **23**, 261–272.

101. Cubilla, A.L., Dilner, J., Schellhammer, P.F., *et al.* (2004) Tumours of the penis: Malignant epithelial tumours. In: *World Health Organization Classification of Tumours. Pathology and Genetics of Tumours of the Urinary System and Male Genital Organs* (eds J.N. Eble, G. Sauter, J.I. Epstein & I.A. Sesterhenn), pp. 281–290. International Agency for Research on Cancer, Lyon.

102. Gerber, G.S. (1994) Carcinoma in situ of the penis. *Journal of Urology*, **151**, 829–833.

103. Patterson, J.W., Kao, G.F., Graham, J.H. & Helwig, E.B. (1986) Bowenoid papulosis. A clinico-pathologic study with ultrastructural observations. *Cancer*, **57**, 823–836.

104. von Krogh, G. & Horenblas, S. (2000) Diagnosis and clinical presentation of premalignant lesions of the penis. *Scandinavian Journal of Urology and Nephrology*, **34**, 201–214.

105. Heideman, D.A., Waterboer, T., Pawlita, M., *et al*. (2007) Human papillomavirus-16 is the predominant type etiologically involved in penile squamous cell carcinoma. *Journal of Clinical Oncology*, **25**, 4550–4556.

106. Pascual, A., Pariente, M., Godinez, J.M., *et al*. (2007) High prevalence of human papillomavirus 16 in penile carcinoma. *Histology and Histopathology*, **22**, 177–183.

107. Carter, J.J., Madeleine, M.M., Shera, K., *et al*. (2001) Human papillomavirus 16 and 18 L1 serology compared across anogenital cancer sites. *Cancer Research*, **61**, 1934–1940.

108. Giuliano, A.R., Lazcano, E., Villa, L.L., *et al*. (2009) Circumcision and sexual behavior: Factors independently associated with human papillomavirus detection among men in the HIM study. *International Journal of Cancer*, **124**, 1251–1257.

109. Gray, R.H., Wawer, M.J., Serwadda, D. & Kigozi, G. (2009) The role of male circumcision in the prevention of human papillomavirus and HIV infection. *Journal of Infectious Diseases*, **199**, 1–3.

110. Kagumire, R. (2008) Ugandan effort to constrain HIV spread hampered by systemic and cultural obstacles to male circumcision. *Canadian Medical Association Journal*, **179**, 1119–1120.

111. Uronis, H.E. & Bendell, J.C. (2007) Anal cancer: An overview. *Oncologist*, **12**, 524–534.

112. Chin-Hong, P.V., Vittinghoff, E., Cranston, R.D., *et al*. (2005) Age-related prevalence of anal cancer precursors in homosexual men: The explore study. *Journal of the National Cancer Institute*, **97**, 896–905.

113. Dunleavey, R. (2005) The role of viruses and sexual transmission in anal cancer. *Nursing Times*, **101**, 38–41.

114. Daling, J.R., Madeleine, M.M., Johnson, L.G., *et al*. (2004) Human papillomavirus, smoking, and sexual practices in the etiology of anal cancer. *Cancer*, **101**, 270–280.

115. Welton, M.L., Sharkey, F.E. & Kahlenberg, M.S. (2004) The etiology and epidemiology of anal cancer. *Surgical Oncology Clinics of North America*, **13**, 263–275.

116. Anderson, J.S., Vajdic, C. & Grulich, A.E. (2004) Is screening for anal cancer warranted in homosexual men? *Sex Health*, **1**, 137–140.

117. Giuliano, A.R., Tortolero-Luna, G., Ferrer, E., *et al*. (2008) Epidemiology of human papillomavirus infection in men, cancers other than cervical and benign conditions. *Vaccine*, **26** (Suppl. 10), K17–K28.

118. Cameron, J.E. & Hagensee, M.E. (2007) Human papillomavirus infection and disease in the HIV+ individual. *Cancer Treatment and Research*, **133**, 185–213.

119. Nyitray, A., Nielson, C.M., Harris, R.B., *et al*. (2008) Prevalence of and risk factors for anal human papillomavirus infection in heterosexual men. *Journal of Infectious Diseases*, **197**, 1676–1684.

120. Kreuter, A. & Wieland, U. (2009) Human papillomavirus-associated diseases in HIV-infected men who have sex with men. *Current Opinion in Infectious Diseases*, **22**, 109–114.

121. Palefsky, J. (2009) Human papillomavirus-related disease in people with HIV. *Current Opinion in HIV and AIDS*, **4**, 52–56.

122. Palefsky, J.M. & Rubin, M. (2009) The epidemiology of anal human papillomavirus and related neoplasia. *Obstetrics Gynecology Clinics of North America*, **36**, 187–200.

123. D'Souza, G., Cook, R.L., Ostrow, D., Johnson-Hill, L.M., Wiley, D. & Silvestre, T. (2008) Anal cancer screening behaviors and intentions in men who have sex with men. *Journal of General Internal Medicine*, **23**, 1452–1457.

124. Gervaz, P., Buchs, N. & Morel, P. (2008) Diagnosis and management of anal cancer. *Current Gastroenterology Reports*, **10**, 502–506.

125. Nadal, S.R., Calore, E.E., Nadal, L.R., Horta, S.H. & Manzione, C.R. (2007) [Anal cytology for screening of pre-neoplasic lesions]. *Revista da Associacao Medica Brasileirs*, **53**, 147–151.

126. Karnon, J., Jones, R., Czoski-Murray, C. & Smith, K.J. (2008) Cost-utility analysis of screening high-risk groups for anal cancer. *Journal of Public Health (Oxford)*, **30**, 293–304.

127. Argiris, A., Karamouzis, M.V., Raben, D. & Ferris, R.L. (2008) Head and neck cancer. *Lancet*, **371**, 1695–1709.

128. Ragin, C.C., Modugno, F. & Gollin, S.M. (2007) The epidemiology and risk factors of head and neck cancer: A focus on human papillomavirus. *Journal of Dental Research*, **86**, 104–114.

129. Marur, S. & Forastiere, A.A. (2008) Head and neck cancer: Changing epidemiology, diagnosis, and treatment. *Mayo Clinic Proceedings*, **83**, 489–501.

130. Herrerro, R., Castelleague, X., Pawlita, M., *et al*. (2003) Human papillomavirus and oral cancer. The International Agency for Research on Cancer multicentre study. *Journal of the National Cancer Institute*, **95**, 1772–1783.

131. Licitra, L., Perrone, F., Bossi, P., *et al*. (2006) High-risk human papillomavirus affects prognosis in patients with surgically treated oropharyngeal squamous cell carcinoma. *Journal of Clinical Oncology*, **24**, 5630–5636.

132. McNeil, C. (2008) Human papillomavirus and oral cancer: Looking toward the clinic. *Journal of National Cancer Institute*, **100**, 840–842.

133. Haraf, D.J., Nodzenski, E., Brachman, D., *et al*. (1996) Human papilloma virus and p53 in head and neck cancer: Clinical correlates and survival. *Clinical Cancer Research*, **2**, 755–762.

134. Ringstrom, E., Peters, E., Hasegawa, M., Posner, M., Liu, M. & Kelsey, K.T. (2002) Human papillomavirus type 16 and squamous cell carcinoma of the head and neck. *Clinical Cancer Research*, **8**, 3187–3192.

135. Psyrri, A. & DiMaio, D. (2008) Human papillomavirus in cervical and head-and-neck cancer. *Nature Clinical Practice Oncology*, **5**, 24–31.

136. Smith, E.M., Ritchie, J.M., Summersgill, K.F., *et al*. (2004) Age, sexual behavior and human papillomavirus infection in oral cavity and oropharyngeal cancers. *International Journal of Cancer*, **108**, 766–772.

137. Hemminki, K., Dong, C. & Frisch, M. (2000) Tonsillar and other upper aerodigestive tract cancers among cervical cancer patients and their husbands. *European Journal of Cancer Prevention*, **9**, 433–437.

138. Schwartz, S.M., Daling, J.R., Doody, D.R., *et al*. (1998) Oral cancer risk in relation to sexual history and evidence of human papillomavirus infection. *Journal of National Cancer Institute*, **90**, 1626–1636.

139. D'Souza, G., Kreimer, A.R., Viscidi, R., *et al*. (2007) Case-control study of human papillomavirus and oropharyngeal cancer. *New England Journal of Medicine*, **356**, 1944–1956.

140. Halpern-Felsher, B.L., Cornell, J.L., Kropp, R.Y. & Tschann, J.M. (2005) Oral versus vaginal sex among adolescents: Perceptions, attitudes, and behavior. *Pediatrics*, **115**, 845–851.

141. Brady, S.S. & Halpern-Felsher, B.L. (2007) Adolescents' reported consequences of having oral sex versus vaginal sex. *Pediatrics*, **119**, 229–236.

142. Ferris, D.G., Waller, J.L., Miller, J., *et al*. (2008) Men's attitudes toward receiving the human papillomavirus vaccine. *Journal of Lower Genital Tract Disease*, **12**, 276–281.

143. Ferris, D.G., Waller, J.L., Miller, J., *et al*. (2009) Variables associated with human papillomavirus (HPV) vaccine acceptance by men. *Journal of the American Board of Family Medicine*, **22**, 34–42.

9 Retroviruses

Certain viruses are unique among known life forms in not having a DNA-based genome; they are known as RNA viruses. A subgroup of RNA viruses, called retroviruses, translates their genome into DNA, using an enzyme called reverse transcriptase, before it is expressed in the host cell. The retrovirus HTLV-1 causes a specific form of T-cell leukaemia/lymphoma in about 5% of those infected; the risk of developing malignancy is influenced by route of infection. Infection with HTLV-1 precedes malignancy by as much as four decades. HIV infection is not directly carcinogenic but the associated immunosuppression increases the risk of all infection-associated malignancies. Highly active anti-retroviral therapy (HAART) reduces the risk of most HIV-linked cancers but not all implying different mechanisms of oncogenesis.

Organisms[1,2]

Retroviruses are so named because they employ an enzyme called reverse transcriptase to translate RNA in a *retro*grade sense – that is, RNA is used as a template to produce DNA. The RNA in retroviruses is known as (+) sense – the sequence runs in the same direction as messenger RNA and could be translated directly to produce a protein – retroviruses do not do this, they translate the RNA into DNA. The DNA intermediate (provirus) integrates into the host genome, where it may remain transcriptionally silent (not be expressed)[3]. The location of integration is random but will always be the same in a given patient[4].

Once viral DNA is integrated into the host genome, if its host cell divides the provirus will be passed to each daughter cell. Because it is not integrated into the DNA of germ cells (sperm, ova) it will not be transmitted to offspring of the infected person. In cases where the provirus is integrated into a germ cell genome, it will be vertically transmitted; although such events are rare, over evolutionary history, this has happened many times and such integrated

Infectious Causes of Cancer, first edition. By Ken Campbell. Published 2011 by John Wiley & Sons Ltd.
© 2011 John Wiley & Sons Ltd.

elements are called (human) *Endogenous RetroViruses* or (h)ERV. It has been estimated that as much as 8% of the human genome consists of heirlooms donated by past viral incursions.[5]

All retroviruses share certain features, unique among viruses;

■ They are the only viruses which are truly diploid
  o They contain two copies of each gene
■ They are the only RNA viruses whose genome is produced by cellular transcriptional machinery
  o They do not produce their own enzymes (polymerases) to do this
■ They are the only viruses whose genome requires a specific cellular RNA (tRNA) for replication
  o All other viruses employ existing cellular tRNA, retroviruses need to produce their own specialized version
■ They are the only (+) sense RNA viruses whose genome does not serve directly as mRNA immediately after infection
  o Other (+) sense RNA viruses use the original viral RNA as a template for protein synthesis, retroviruses first generate a DNA copy, which is integrated into the host genome and codes for mRNA in the usual manner

All retroviruses contain three genes, in an invariant order, *gag*, *pol* and *env*[1]; *gag* encodes for internal structural proteins of the virus, *pol* encodes for the enzyme retroviral transcriptase and for the enzyme which integrates viral DNA into the host genome, and *env* encodes for the envelope proteins which make the viral capsule[1]. Many retroviruses contain additional genes; this is true for both of the human oncogenic retroviruses, HTLV-1 and HIV[6]. Retroviruses target the centrosome, an organelle which plays a vital role in cell division[7]; it is not yet clear whether this is significant for oncogenesis.

Human T-cell lymphotropic virus 1 (HTLV-1)
(*Synonym* – Human T-cell leukaemia virus 1)
The designation lymphotropic is preferred because the lymphoid malignancy caused by the virus typically presents with mixed features of both leukaemia and lymphoma – adult T-cell leukaemia/lymphoma (ATLL)[8]. ATLL was first described in 1977 in people living in Southern Japan; it was originally know as adult T-cell leukaemia (ATL), which reflects the prevalence of leukaemic features in the Japanese population[9]. HTLV was first isolated by Robert Gallo, from malignant T cells of a 28-year black American male with cutaneous lymphoma[10], by 1982 it had been shown that this was specifically tropic to T cells[11] and that the virus is present in almost all cases of the malignancy[12].

Professor Danny Catovsky noted the comparably high prevalence of T cell malignancies among Caribbean immigrants living in London. Catovsky noted the clinical similarity between this and the Japanese cases and speculated that this was one and the same disease. He invited Robert Gallo to a meeting with fellow haematologists, virologists, molecular biologists and epidemiologists;

this led to a targeted study in the Caribbean which confirmed Catovsky's suspicion – it was found that endemicity in certain Caribbean islands was related to the African tribes from which the population had descended[13,14]. Most cases seen in the UK are in people of Afro-Caribbean descent, although it is also seen in the white population[15].

There are three main subfamilies of the retrovirus family, *'the RNA tumour viruses (oncovirinae); the "slow" viruses (lentivirinae); and the "foamy" viruses (spumavirinae)'*[16]; HTLV belongs to the oncovirinae and is further sub-classified as C-type[13]. There are other closely related HTLV types but none of these has been classed by International Agency for Research on Cancer (IARC) as being definitely, or even possibly, carcinogenic to humans. This leaves a one-to-one relationship, with HTLV-1 as the only defined carcinogenic type and ATLL as the only malignancy defined as being caused by an HTLV type[17,18]. The geographical distribution of HTLV-1 is striking, with limited endemic areas within Japan, Africa, the Caribbean islands and South America, and low numbers of cases are seen in countries with immigration from these places[19]. There are estimated to be around 15–20 million infected persons worldwide[20]; there is no satisfactory explanation as to why the disease is common in one area, such as south-western Japan and yet almost completely absent from neighbouring regions of Korea, China and Eastern Russia or for isolated pockets such as those in Iran[19].

In some areas, such as the Caribbean islands, this may reflect the origins of the affected populations, for example the areas in Africa from which the present population derive[21].

Transmission is by three routes, blood-borne (the most efficient), sexual transmission (particularly male to female) and vertical (chiefly by breast-feeding)[22]. As viraemia is minimal or absent, cell-free body fluids cannot cause infection – this requires transfer of infected lymphocytes[23]. It has been reported that male to female transmission is more common, which would be consistent with need for transfer of infected cells, but other reports have questioned this[24,25]. The discrepancy may be related to observed differences in risk of male to female transmission related to whether the male partner has antibodies to the HTLV-1 *tax* gene[26]. In endemic areas vertical transmission is by far the most common, especially when breast feeding is prolonged beyond 3 months; *'Rates of transmission from mother to child are 2.7% in formula fed infants, 5% with three months' breast feeding, and up to 20% with prolonged breast feeding'*[27]. In these populations latency between infection and development of ATL is typically decades long and the rate of malignant disease is only around 1%–3% of those infected[28]. Latency varies between endemic areas, with onset being later in Japan than in Brazil, for example[29] – it has been suggested that this is because parasite infection may modulate the progression of HTLV-induced disease[30,31].

HTLV-1 infection is rare in the indigenous population of Western Europe, with most cases occurring in migrants from endemic areas. In the past the most common mode of transmission in non-endemic countries was transfusion of contaminated blood[32-34]. Animal studies indicated that as little as 0.01 ml of virus-infected blood can transmit HTLV; epidemiological studies indicate that ATLL may occur following transfusion and there may be a higher probability of aggressive disease and a very much shorter latency in this context[35,36].

Many countries have now introduced routine screening of blood donations for HTLV[36-40]. The UK now routinely screens all units and the risk, in the UK, of transfusional infection is now close to zero[41]. A significant minority of cases occurs in i.v. drug users but it is plausible that this group will have a low incidence of ATLL, based on the evidence for low risk of ATLL following horizontal transmission. In 2005 an analysis was published of Health Protection Agency (HPA) data on new cases of HTLV infection in England and Wales between 2002 and 2004[42]; there were a total of 273 cases, with a majority of cases being of black Caribbean ethnicity, about 90% of cases were either vertically transmitted (mother to child) or acquired by heterosexual intercourse. Based on data from 1987 onwards, it appears that incidence peaked in 2003; probably because of identification of infected individuals within the blood donor pool[43], diagnoses now continue at a stable level of about 90 cases per year. A 2009 European survey indicated that the UK incidence in first time blood donors is on the order of 5 in 100 000[40].

HTLV infection is also established as the cause of a debilitating progressive neurological disorder called HTLV-I associated myelopathy/tropical spastic paraparesis (HAM/TSP)[44,45]. Both experimental and epidemiological evidence indicate that vertical transmission is associated with both ATLL and HAM/TSP, whereas horizontal transmission causes HAM/TSP but is not linked with lymphoid malignancy[46,47]; it is thought that this is because vertical transmission leads to *'insufficient HTLV-I-specific T-cell response and expansion of infected cells'*[48].

Human immunodeficiency virus[49-52]

The human immunodeficiency virus (HIV) is a lentivirus (lenti – slow), which induces profound immunosuppression in infected individuals. Typical features of lentivirus infection are[53]:

■ Chronic course of disease
■ A long period of clinical latency
■ Persistent viral replication
■ Involvement of the central nervous system

The UN Global report on HIV/AIDS 2008[50] offers some truly staggering estimates of the scale of the epidemic, *'In 2007 alone, 33 million [30 million–36 million] people were living with HIV, 2.7 million [2.2 million–3.2 million] people became infected with the virus, and 2 million [1.8 million–2.3 million] people died of HIV-related causes'.* [The figures in brackets represent the upper and lower limits of estimates.] In an update published in November 2009[54] the figures (with error margins) were as follows:

■ People living with HIV 33.4 million (31.1 – 35.8 m)
■ People becoming infected with HIV 2.7 million (2.4–3.0 m)
■ Deaths from HIV-related causes 2.0 million (1.7–2.4 m)

Perhaps the key sentence from the update is, '*The latest epidemiological data indicate that globally the spread of HIV appears to have peaked in 1996, when 3.5 million [3.2 million–3.8 million] new HIV infections occurred. In 2008, the estimated number of new HIV infections was approximately 30% lower than at the epidemic's peak 12 years earlier*'. This was widely reported as AIDS being on the decline; as the authors make clear, the incidence continued to rise but at a slower rate.

An excellent free textbook on HIV / AIDS is available as a download from http:// www.hivmedicine.com/. The discussion in this section will be confined to those aspects which are relevant to malignant disease. There is no evidence that HIV acts as a direct or even indirect carcinogen. The association with infection-associated cancer is a consequence of its immunosuppressive effects. An important distinction is drawn between infection with HIV and AIDS; this is based on the presence or absence of AIDS-defining illness[55]:

- Candidiasis of bronchi, trachea or lungs
- Candidiasis, oesophageal
- **Cervical cancer, invasive**
- Coccidioidomycosis, disseminated or extrapulmonary
- Cryptococcosis, extrapulmonary
- Cryptosporidiosis, chronic intestinal (greater than 1 month's duration)
- Cytomegalovirus disease (other than liver, spleen or nodes)
- Cytomegalovirus retinitis (with loss of vision)
- Encephalopathy, HIV-related
- Herpes simplex: chronic ulcer(s) (greater than 1 month's duration); or bronchitis, pneumonitis or oesophagitis
- Histoplasmosis, disseminated or extrapulmonary
- Isosporiasis, chronic intestinal (greater than 1 month's duration)
- **Kaposi's sarcoma**
- **Lymphoma, Burkitt's (or equivalent term)**
- **Lymphoma, immunoblastic (or equivalent)**
- **Lymphoma, primary, of brain**
- *Mycobacterium avium* complex or *M. kansasii*, disseminated or extrapulmonary
- *Mycobacterium tuberculosis*, any site (pulmonary or extrapulmonary)
- Mycobacterium, other species or unidentified species, disseminated or extrapulmonary
- Pneumocystis pneumonia
- Progressive multifocal leukoencephalopathy
- Salmonella septicemia, recurrent
- Toxoplasmosis of brain
- Wasting syndrome due to HIV

Malignant neoplasms shown in **bold**

Although only these cancers are part of the AIDS definition, there are several others which are seen at increased frequency in HIV positive individuals.

The introduction of combinations of anti-retroviral drugs, known as Highly Active Anti-Retroviral Therapy (HAART), has led to a marked reduction in the incidence of AIDS-defining illnesses in treated patients[56,57]. Unfortunately, for many of the populations of countries most affected by HIV/AIDS HAART is totally unaffordable and HIV continues to be followed inevitably by AIDS and death[50].

The epidemiology and transmission of HIV is now very well known; the routes of transmission are[55]:

- Unprotected sexual intercourse with an infected partner
- Injection or transfusion of contaminated blood or blood products (infection through artificial insemination, skin grafts and organ transplants is also possible)
- Sharing unsterilized injection equipment that has been previously used by someone who is infected
- Maternofoetal transmission (during pregnancy, at birth, and through breast-feeding)

HIV cannot be transmitted by casual social contact, sharing of eating utensils or crockery or by tears or saliva (unless contaminated with blood) – most experts concur that it cannot be spread by contact of blood with intact undamaged skin. Although there has been speculation that it might be spread by blood-sucking insects or mammals, there is no evidence that this has ever actually occurred[55].

Worryingly, despite overwhelming scientific consensus there are still many who not only deny the link between HIV and AIDS but vigorously proselytize in favour of their position[58].

Associated malignancies

Human T-cell lymphotropic virus 1 (HTLV-1)

Adult T-cell leukaemia/lymphoma[22,23,59–61]
HTLV-1 is the causal agent for Adult T-cell Leukaemia/Lymphoma – ATLL, which is a lymphoid malignancy first described in a series of 16 Japanese patients in 1977[9]. The final sentence of the seminal paper presciently stated, 'Genetic background may play an important role but other factors such as oncogenic virus infections must be explored'.

The manner in which HTLV induces ATLL is not fully understood; however expression of the viral tax gene is believed to be both necessary and sufficient for oncogenesis[62]. It has been shown that HTLV-1 tax expression leads to altered function of the centrosome, which is a key structure involved in cell division[7]. Although both CD4 and CD8 T cells are susceptible to infection with HTLV, ATLL almost exclusively exhibits a CD4 phenotype; it has been proposed that this selectivity is related to differences in tax activity between T cell subtypes[63,64].

There are four subtypes of ATLL, smouldering, chronic and two acute forms known as leukaemic and lymphomatous[59]

1. Smoldering ATLL
   - Atypical lymphocytes
   - Limited skin lesions
2. Chronic ATLL
   - Lymphocytosis
   - Skin lesions
   - Liver, lung, lymph node involvement
3. Acute ATLL – lymphomatous form
   - T-cell non-Hodgkin's lymphoma
   - Frequent blood, skin, bone lesions
4. Acute ATLL – leukaemia form
   - T-cell leukaemia
   - Hypercalcemia
   - Lytic bone lesions
   - Lymphadenopathy
   - Visceral or leptomeningeal involvement
   - Opportunistic infections

Cofactors

There are no definite cofactors for ATLL, although it has been proposed that co-infection with *Strongyloides stercoralis* may be associated with a shortened latency[30,31].

Prevention

ATLL is rare in the developed world, and may remain so, even in the face of increases in horizontally acquired infections. It will be decades before the impact of adult-acquired infection on the incidence of ATLL can be directly assessed but there is evidence to suggest it will be minimal. The North Thames neonatal screening laboratory estimated, in 2003, that '*An estimated 223 (95% confidence interval 110–350) of the 720 000 pregnant women each year in the United Kingdom are infected with HTLV*'[27]. Although it was recommended over 15 years ago that neonatal screening would be cost-effective[65], this is still not current practice.

In endemic areas, recommendations to bottle feed, or at least to shorten duration of breast-feeding have had a significant impact on incidence. In the UK, neonates whose mothers were born in the Caribbean had a seroprevalence of 17 per 1000; comparable with that for HIV[27].

Human immunodeficiency virus (HIV)

Table 9.1 illustrates the relative risk of certain cancers in persons with HIV/AIDS.

Table 9.1 Relative risk of certain cancers in persons with HIV/AIDS (Based on data from Ref.[66]).

Cancer	Causal agent	RR for men	RR for women
Kaposi sarcoma	**HHV-8**	**98**	**203**
NHL	**EBV/HHV-8**	**37**	**55**
Cervical (invasive)	HPV		9
HL	EBV	8	6
Tongue	HPV/EBV	2	7
Rectal/anal	HPV (anal carcinoma)	3	3
Liver (primary)	HCV, HBV, alcohol	5	
CNS	EBV (CNS 1° lymphoma)	3	3
Skin (excluding KS)	HPV, UV light	21	8

Source: Reprinted by permission from Macmillan Publishers Ltd: *Nature Reviews Cancer*, copyright (2002). *Note*: AIDS-defining cancers are shown in **bold**.

AIDS-defining malignancies[67]

The US Center for Disease Control (CDC) defines three groups of malignancies as AIDS-defining; Kaposi sarcoma, certain forms of non-Hodgkin's lymphoma and invasive cervical cancer. Although not AIDS-defining, cervical dysplasia (moderate or severe) or cervical carcinoma in situ are defined as HIV-related symptomatic conditions, that is, they are considered to reflect progression of the HIV infection towards AIDS.

Non-AIDS-defining malignancies[66]

There are certain cancers, which although not considered by CDC to be AIDS-defining, are seen more frequently in HIV positive individuals. These are cancers of the tongue, anorectal cancer, primary liver cancer, primary cancer of the central nervous system and cancers of the skin, excluding Kaposi sarcoma (which is AIDS-defining)[66].

Cofactors

In cases where it is associated with an increased cancer risk, HIV infection appears to act as a cofactor, rather than a primary cause.

Prevention[68]

A striking phenomenon observed since the introduction of HAART has been a reduced incidence of AIDS-defining cancers in treated individuals, coupled with an increase in the incidence of non-AIDS-defining cancers[69–71]. Non-AIDS-defining cancers in the HAART cohort were associated with increasing age and white race, reflecting the strong contribution of skin cancer[69]. Although the introduction of HAART has extended survival of people with HIV or AIDS (PWHA) in the developed world, it has had little impact in the countries most devastated by the AIDS epidemic. Of the AIDS-defining cancers, perhaps the greatest hope in the short term is for a reduction of cervical cancer by introduction of vaccination.

Despite 25 years of research and billions of dollars of investment, it appears that a vaccine against HIV is as far away as ever[72,73]. While this remains the case, the focus on AIDS control will continue to be on programmes to prevent spread of the virus. The most hopeful results so far are from ABC campaigns (*Abstain, Be* faithful, use a *Condom*) and campaigns to reduce or eliminate mother-to-child transmission[74]. Unfortunately, only a minority of governments are acting decisively to reduce transmission of blood-borne/sexually transmitted infections in prisons[75].

It is to be regretted that, when condom use has been shown so emphatically to reduce the risk of HIV transmission, the leader of the Catholic Church should suggest that condom use aggravates the problem[76]; it has been suggested that the Church, within its existing dogma, could accept prophylactic (disease prevention) use of condoms, while continuing to proscribe their use for contraception[77]. There is some hope within the US healthcare community that President Obama will discard the Bush administrations emphasis on 'abstinence only' campaigns, in favour of the ABC approach, which has proved objectively more effective[78].

One measure for which there is strong evidence is male circumcision[79], this may also offer protection against HPV infection but this appears only true if carried out at an early stage[80]. It is possible that male circumcision may be less acceptable in some high risk populations than others[81]. A 2010 review concluded that, '*Safe, high quality, low cost adult male circumcision services should be made available to regions with a high HIV incidence as part of a comprehensive HIV prevention package*'[82].

Summary

■ Retroviruses are RNA viruses which must translate their genome into DNA, using an enzyme called reverse transcriptase, before it can be expressed in the host cell
■ HTLV-1 is the only directly carcinogenic retrovirus
  o HTLV-1 infection is associated with a specific form of T-cell leukaemia/lymphoma in about 5% of those infected
  o Risk of developing malignancy is influenced by route of infection
  o Infection precedes malignancy by as much as 4 decades
■ HIV infection is not directly carcinogenic
  o The associated immunosuppression increases the risk of all infection-associated malignancies

○ HAART reduces the risk of most HIV-linked cancers but not all

○ In certain instances, for example cervical cancer, co-infection with HIV increases the risk of progression of precursor lesions to frank malignancy

Infection with HTLV-1 retrovirus is associated with one specific cancer, while HIV infection is not directly carcinogenic but does increase the risk of all infection-associated cancers. HTLV-1 is rare in the UK population and is seen almost exclusively in migrants from endemic areas. The virus is often vertically transmitted so it is valuable for healthcare staff in obstetric practice to be aware of its existence and of the advice which should be given to minimize risk of transmission.

HIV infection is much more common than HTLV-1 in the UK population. Recent data indicate that the rate of spread of HIV is slowing, although numbers of cases will continue to increase for some time. Any person who is known to be HIV-positive should be advised on the need for particular care to minimize their risk of infections associated with cancer. HAART has been shown to reduce the risk of AIDS-defining cancer in PWA; a significant minority of PWA are reluctant to take anti-retroviral therapy due to toxicity – it may be helpful to inform them of the protection afforded against cancer[58].

References

1. Balvay, L., Lopez-Lastra, M., Sargueil, B., Darlix, J.L. & Ohlmann, T. (2007) Translational control of retroviruses. *Nature Reviews Microbiology*, **5**, 128–140.

2. Goff, S.P. (2007) Host factors exploited by retroviruses. *Nature Reviews Microbiology*, **5**, 253–263.

3. Gallo, R.C. (1995) Human retroviruses in the second decade: A personal perspective. *Nature Medicine*, **1**, 753–759.

4. Yoshida, M. (1999) Human C-type oncoviruses and T-cell leukaemia/lymphoma. In: *Microbes and Malignancy: Infection as a Cause of Human Cancers* (ed. J. Parsonnet), pp. 289–309. OUP, Oxford.

5. Weiss, R.A. (2006) The discovery of endogenous retroviruses. *Retrovirology*, **3**, 67.

6. Weiss, R.A. (2001) Retroviruses and cancer. *Current Science*, **81**, 528–534.

7. Afonso, P.V., Zamborlini, A., Saib, A. & Mahieux, R. (2007) Centrosome and retroviruses: The dangerous liaisons. *Retrovirology*, **4**, 27.

8. Dahmoush, L., Hijazi, Y., Barnes, E., Stetler-Stevenson, M. & Abati, A. (2002) Adult T-cell leukemia/lymphoma: A cytopathologic, immunocytochemical, and flow cytometric study. *Cancer*, **96**, 110–116.

9. Uchiyama, T., Yodoi, J., Sagawa, K., Takatsuki, K. & Uchino, H. (1977) Adult T-cell leukemia: Clinical and hematologic features of 16 cases. *Blood*, **50**, 481–492.

10. Poiesz, B.J., Ruscetti, F.W., Gazdar, A.F., Bunn, P.A., Minna, J.D. & Gallo, R.C. (1980) Detection and isolation of type C retrovirus particles from fresh and cultured lymphocytes of a patient with cutaneous T-cell lymphoma. *Proceedings of the National Academy of Sciences of the United States of America*, **77**, 7415–7419.

11. Gallo, R.C., Mann, D., Broder, S., *et al.* (1982) Human T-cell leukemia-lymphoma virus (HTLV) is in T but not B lymphocytes from a patient with cutaneous T-cell lymphoma. *Proceedings of the National Academy of Sciences of the Unites States of America*, **79**, 5680–5683.

12. Kalyanaraman, V.S., Sarngadharan, M.G., Nakao, Y., Ito, Y., Aoki, T. & Gallo, R.C. (1982) Natural antibodies to the structural core protein (p24) of the human T-cell leukemia (lymphoma) retrovirus found in sera of leukemia patients in Japan. *Proceedings of National Academy Sciences of the United States of America*, **79**, 1653–1657.

13. Blattner, W.A., Kalyanaraman, V.S., Robert-Guroff, M., *et al.* (1982) The human type-C retrovirus, HTLV, in Blacks from the Caribbean region, and relationship to adult T-cell leukemia/lymphoma. *International Journal of Cancer*, **30**, 257–264.

14. Gallo, R.C., Kalyanaraman, V.S., Sarngadharan, M.G., *et al.* (1983) Association of the human type C retrovirus with a subset of adult T-cell cancers. *Cancer Research*, **43**, 3892–3899.

15. Dougan, S., Smith, A., Tosswill, J.C., Davison, K., Zuckerman, M. & Taylor, G.P. (2005) New diagnoses of HTLV infection in England and Wales: 2002–2004. *Eurosurveillance*, **10**, 232–235.

16. Weiss, R.A. (1987) Retroviruses and human disease. *Journal of Clinical Pathology*, **40**, 1064–1069.

17. IARC (1996) Human immunodeficiency viruses and human T-cell lymphotropic viruses. *IARC Monographs on the Evaluation of Carcinogenic Risks to Humans*, **67**, 31–38. International Agency for Research on Cancer, Lyon.

18. Verdonck, K., Gonzalez, E., Van Dooren, S., Vandamme, A.M., Vanham, G. & Gotuzzo, E. (2007) Human T-lymphotropic virus 1: Recent knowledge of an ancient infection. *Lancet Infectious Disease*, **7**, 266–281.

19. Proietti, F.A., Carneiro-Proietti, A.B., Catalan-Soares, B.C. & Murphy, E.L. (2005) Global epidemiology of HTLV-I infection and associated diseases. *Oncogene*, **24**, 6058–6068.

20. De The, G. & Kazanji, M. (1996) An HTLV-I/II vaccine: From animal models to clinical trials? *Journal of Acquired Immune Deficiency Syndrome and Human Retrovirology*, **13** (Suppl. 1), S191–S198.

21. Vidal, A.U., Gessain, A., Yoshida, M., *et al.* (1994) Phylogenetic classification of human T cell leukaemia/lymphoma virus type I genotypes in five major molecular and geographical subtypes. *Journal of General Virology*, **75** (Pt 12), 3655–3666.

22. Manns, A., Hisada, M. & La Grenade, L. (1999) Human T-lymphotropic virus type I infection. *Lancet*, **353**, 1951–1958.

23. Neely, S.M. (1989) Adult T-cell leukemia-lymphoma. *Western Journal of Medicine*, **150**, 557–561.

24. Figueroa, J.P., Ward, E., Morris, J., *et al.* (1997) Incidence of HIV and HTLV-1 infection among sexually transmitted disease clinic attenders in Jamaica. *Journal of Acquired Immune Deficiency Syndrome and Human Retrovirology*, **15**, 232–237.

25. Roucoux, D.F., Wang, B., Smith, D., *et al.* (2005) A prospective study of sexual transmission of human T lymphotropic virus (HTLV)-I and HTLV-II. *Journal of Infectious Disease*, **191**, 1490–1497.

26. Chen, Y.M., Okayama, A., Lee, T.H., Tachibana, N., Mueller, N. & Essex, M. (1991) Sexual transmission of human T-cell leukemia virus type I associated with the presence of anti-Tax antibody. *Proceedings of the National Academy of Sciences of the United States of America*, **88**, 1182–1186.

27. Ades, A.E., Parker, S., Walker, J., Edginton, M., Taylor, G.P. & Weber, J.N. (2000) Human T cell leukaemia/lymphoma virus infection in pregnant women in the United Kingdom: Population study. *BMJ*, **320**, 1497–1501.

28. Cleghorn, F.R., Manns, A., Falk, R., *et al.* (1995) Effect of human T-lymphotropic virus type I infection on non-Hodgkin's lymphoma incidence. *Journal of the National Cancer Institute*, **87**, 1009–1014.

29. Pombo De Oliveira, M.S., Matutes, E., Schulz, T., *et al.* (1995) T-cell malignancies in Brazil. Clinico-pathological and molecular studies of HTLV-I-positive and -negative cases. *International Journal of Cancer*, **60**, 823–827.

30. Gabet, A.S., Mortreux, F., Talarmin, A., *et al.* (2000) High circulating proviral load with oligoclonal expansion of HTLV-1 bearing T cells in HTLV-1 carriers with strongyloidiasis. *Oncogene*, **19**, 4954–4960.

31. Satoh, M., Toma, H., Sugahara, K., *et al.* (2002) Involvement of IL-2/IL-2R system activation by parasite antigen in polyclonal expansion of CD4(+)25(+) HTLV-1-infected T-cells in human carriers of both HTLV-1 and S. stercoralis. *Oncogene*, **21**, 2466–2475.

32. Okochi, K., Sato, H. & Hinuma, Y. (1984) A retrospective study on transmission of adult T cell leukemia virus by blood transfusion: Seroconversion in recipients. *Vox Sanguinis*, **46**, 245–253.

33. Okochi, K. & Sato, H. (1984) Transmission of ATLV (HTLV-I) through blood transfusion. *Princess Takamatsu Symposium*, **15**, 129–135.

34. (1991) Public Health Service inter-agency guidelines for screening donors of blood, plasma, organs, tissues, and semen for evidence of hepatitis B and hepatitis C. *MMWR Recommendations and Reports*, **40**, 1–17.

35. Chen, Y.C., Wang, C.H., Su, I.J., *et al.* (1989) Infection of human T-cell leukemia virus type I and development of human T-cell leukemia lymphoma in patients with hematologic neoplasms: A possible linkage to blood transfusion. *Blood*, **74**, 388–394.

36. Osame, M., Izumo, S., Igata, A., *et al.* (1986) Blood transfusion and HTLV-I associated myelopathy. *Lancet*, **2**, 104–105.

37. Taylor, G.P. (1996) The epidemiology of HTLV-I in Europe. *Journal of Acquired Immune Deficiency Syndrome and Human Retrovirology*, **13** (Suppl. 1), S8–S14.

38. Brennan, M., Runganga, J., Barbara, J.A., *et al.* (1993) Prevalence of antibodies to human T cell leukaemia/lymphoma virus in blood donors in north London. *BMJ*, **307**, 1235–1239.

39. Pennington, J., Taylor, G.P., Sutherland, J., *et al.* (2002) Persistence of HTLV-I in blood components after leukocyte depletion. *Blood*, **100**, 677–681.

40. Laperche, S., Worms, B. & Pillonel, J. (2009) Blood safety strategies for human T-cell lymphotropic virus in Europe. *Vox Sanguinis*, **96**, 104–110.

41. Regan, F.A., Hewitt, P., Barbara, J.A. & Contreras, M. (2000) Prospective investigation of transfusion transmitted infection in recipients of over 20 000 units of blood. TTI Study Group. *BMJ*, **320**, 403–406.

42. Dorweiler, I.J., Ruone, S.J., Wang, H., Burry, R.W. & Mansky, L.M. (2006) Role of the human T-cell leukemia virus type 1 PTAP motif in Gag targeting and particle release. *Journal of Virology*, **80**, 3634–3643.

43. Payne, L.J., Tosswill, J.H., Taylor, G.P., Zuckerman, M. & Simms, I. (2004) In the shadow of HIV-HTLV infection in England and Wales, 1987–2001. *Communicable Disease and Public Health*, **7**, 200–206.

44. Osame, M., Usuku, K., Izumo, S., *et al.* (1986) HTLV-I associated myelopathy, a new clinical entity. *Lancet*, **1**, 1031–1032.

45. Gessain, A., Barin, F., Vernant, J.C., *et al.* (1985) Antibodies to human T-lymphotropic virus type-I in patients with tropical spastic paraparesis. *Lancet*, **2**, 407–410.

46. Hasegawa, A., Ohashi, T., Hanabuchi, S., *et al.* (2003) Expansion of human T-cell leukemia virus type 1 (HTLV-1) reservoir in orally infected rats: Inverse correlation with HTLV-1-specific cellular immune response. *Journal of Virology*, **77**, 2956–2963.

47. Kato, H., Koya, Y., Ohashi, T., *et al.* (1998) Oral administration of human T-cell leukemia virus type 1 induces immune unresponsiveness with persistent infection in adult rats. *Journal of Virology*, **72**, 7289–7293.

48. Kannagi, M., Harashima, N., Kurihara, K., *et al.* (2005) Tumor immunity against adult T-cell leukemia. *Cancer Science*, **96**, 249–255.

49. Hoffman, C., Rockstroh, J. & Kamps, B.S. (2007) *HIV Medicine 2007*. Flying Publisher, Paris.

50. UNAIDS (2008) Report on the global HIV/AIDS epidemic 2008.

51. Simon, V., Ho, D.D. & Abdool Karim Q. (2006) HIV/AIDS epidemiology, pathogenesis, prevention, and treatment. *Lancet*, **368**, 489–504.

52. Volberding, P.A., Baker, K.R. & Levine, A.M. (2003) Human immunodeficiency virus hematology. *Hematology (American Society of Hematology Education Program Book)*, **1**, 294–313.

53. Rubbert, A., Behrens, G. & Ostrowski, M. (2007) Pathogenesis of HIV-1 infection. In: *HIV Medicine 2007*(eds C. Hoffman, J.K. Rockstroh & B. Kamps), pp. 59–86. Flying Publisher, Paris.

54. UNAIDS/WHO (2009) AIDS epidemic update: November 2009.

55. Kamps, B.S. & Hoffman, C. (2007) Introduction. In: *HIV Medicine 2007* (eds C. Hoffman, J.K. Rockstroh & B.S. Kamps), pp. 23–32. Flying Publisher, Paris.

56. Palella, F.J., Jr., Delaney, K.M., Moorman, A.C., *et al.* (1998) Declining morbidity and mortality among patients with advanced human immunodeficiency virus infection. HIV outpatient study investigators. *New England Journal of Medicine*, **338**, 853–860.

57. Levine, A.M., Hancock, B.W., MacPhail, P., Ruff, P. & Ashcroft, R.E. (2003) The treatment of AIDS-related cancers. *Lancet Oncology*, **4**, 576–581.

58. Sharp, R. (1 Dec. 2009) A disease of the mind *Independent*; Independent Life, 2–5.

59. Ratner, L. (2005) Human T cell lymphotropic virus-associated leukemia/lymphoma. *Current Opinion in Oncology*, **17**, 469–473.

60. Takatsuki, K. (1984) Adult T-cell leukemia/lymphoma (ATL). *Japanese Journal of Medicine*, **23**, 81–83.

61. Takatsuki, K. (1995) Adult T-cell leukemia. *Internal Medicine*, **34**, 947–952.

62. Bogenberger, J. & Laybourn, P. (2008) Human T lymphotropic virus type 1 protein Tax reduces histone levels. *Retrovirology*, **5**, 9.

63. Semmes, O.J. (2006) Adult T cell leukemia: A tale of two T cells. *Journal of linical Investigation*, **116**, 858–860.

64. Sibon, D., Gabet, A.S., Zandecki, M., *et al.* (2006) HTLV-1 propels untransformed CD4 lymphocytes into the cell cycle while protecting CD8 cells from death. *Journal of Clinical Investigation*, **116**, 974–983.

65. Pagliuca, A., Pawson, R. & Mufti, G.J. (1995) HTLV-I screening in Britain. *BMJ*, **311**, 1313–1314.

66. Boshoff, C. & Weiss, R. (2002) AIDS-related malignancies. *Nature Reviews Cancer*, **2**, 373–382.

67. Centers for Disease Control (1993) 1993 Revised classification system for HIV infection and expanded surveillance case definition for AIDS among adolescents and adults. *Morbidity Mortality Weekly Report*, **42**, RR17.

68. Al Jabri, A.A. & Alenzi, F.Q. (2009) Vaccines, virucides and drugs against HIV/AIDS: Hopes and optimisms for the future. *Open AIDS Journal*, **3**, 1–3.

69. Crum-Cianflone, N., Hullsiek, K.H., Marconi, V., *et al.* (2009) Trends in the incidence of cancers among HIV-infected persons and the impact of antiretroviral therapy: A 20-year cohort study. *AIDS*, **23**, 41–50.

70. Long, J.L., Engels, E.A., Moore, R.D. & Gebo, K.A. (2008) Incidence and outcomes of malignancy in the HAART era in an urban cohort of HIV-infected individuals. *AIDS*, **22**, 489–496.

71. Burgi, A., Brodine, S., Wegner, S., *et al.* (2005) Incidence and risk factors for the occurrence of non-AIDS-defining cancers among human immunodeficiency virus-infected individuals. *Cancer*, **104**, 1505–1511.

72. Cohen, M.S., Hellmann, N., Levy, J.A., DeCock, K. & Lange, J. (2008) The spread, treatment, and prevention of HIV-1: Evolution of a global pandemic. *Journal of Clinical Investigators*, **118**, 1244–1254.

73. Virgin, H.W. & Walker, B.D. (2010) Immunology and the elusive AIDS vaccine. *Nature*, **464**, 224–231.

74. United Nations Children's Fund (UNICEF). (2008) Children and AIDS: Second stocktaking report.

75. Elliott, R. (2007) Deadly disregard: Government refusal to implement evidence-based measures to prevent HIV and hepatitis C virus infections in prisons. *CMAJ*, **177**, 262–264.

76. Roehr, B. (2009) Pope claims that condoms exacerbate HIV and AIDS problem. *BMJ*, **338**, b1206.

77. Kamerow, D. (2009) The papal position on condoms and HIV. *BMJ*, **338**, b1217.

78. Hawes, S.E., Sow, P.S. & Kiviat, N.B. (2007) Is there a role for abstinence only programmes for HIV prevention in high income countries? *BMJ*, **335**, 217–218.

79. Auvert, B., Taljaard, D., Lagarde, E., Sobngwi-Tambekou, J., Sitta, R. & Puren, A. (2005) Randomized, controlled intervention trial of male circumcision for reduction of HIV infection risk: The ANRS 1265 trial. *PLoS Medicine*, **2**, e298.

80. Daling, J.R., Madeleine, M.M., Johnson, L.G., *et al.* (2005) Penile cancer: Importance of circumcision, human papillomavirus and smoking in in situ and invasive disease. *International Journal of Cancer* **116**, 606–616.

81. Kagumire, R. (2008) Ugandan effort to constrain HIV spread hampered by systemic and cultural obstacles to male circumcision. *CMAJ*, **179**, 1119–1120.

82. Doyle, S.M., Kahn, J.G., Hosang, N. & Carroll, P.R. (2010) The impact of male circumcision on HIV transmission. *Journal of Urology*, **183**(1), 21–26.

10 Polyomaviruses

There has been widespread discussion of the possible role of polyomaviruses in human cancers but no polyomavirus has been confirmed as a human carcinogen[1-4]. Merkel cell polyomavirus has recently been described and has a strong, potentially causal, relationship with Merkel cell carcinoma of the skin. There has been widespread speculation about the carcinogenic potential of SV 40 polyomavirus; International Agency for Research on Cancer (IARC) currently does not classify SV 40 as carcinogenic, so it is described here for the sake of completeness.

SV 40 is a simian polyomavirus; prior to the mid-twentieth century there may have been sporadic transfer between its natural host and humans. In 1960, the virus was first isolated from contaminated polio vaccine. By the time precautionary measures had been taken it was estimated that millions of doses of SV 40 containing vaccine had been administered. Subsequently, it was reported that SV 40 had been isolated from human cancers, including mesothelioma.

Organisms

Polyomaviridae were originally included within a wider family called papovaviridae, along with papillomaviridae; the family was split on the basis of marked sequence differences[5]. Polyomaviruses are small viruses with a double-stranded DNA genome and no envelope. There are two clearly pathogenic human strains, called BK and JC from the initials of the index patients; BK may cause polyomavirus nephropathy[6] and JC may cause progressive multifocal leukoencephalopathy[7]. BK and JC virus establish life-long, silent infections in healthy individuals but can become reactivated if the host becomes immunosuppressed.

Simian virus 40 (SV 40)

SV 40 is a simian virus not naturally found in humans; it was introduced to the human population in batches of contaminated polio vaccine[8]. In the early 1960s there were several reports that SV 40 was capable of inducing tumours in animals

Infectious Causes of Cancer, first edition. By Ken Campbell. Published 2011 by John Wiley & Sons Ltd.
© 2011 John Wiley & Sons Ltd.

and malignant transformation in tissue culture[9–16]; a recent report has reviewed the evidence on SV 40 cell transforming and oncogenic potential[17]. In 1992, Bergsagel and colleagues reported the detection of SV 40-like DNA sequences in paediatric tumours[18]; one of the tumour types (ependomyomas) had previously been induced in hamsters by SV 40 injection[13].

In response to the concerns raised, the US Institute of Medicine carried out an immunization safety review of 'SV 40 contamination of polio vaccine and cancer'[19]. The conclusion was that '*The committee concludes that the evidence is inadequate to accept or reject a causal relationship between SV 40-containing polio vaccines and cancer*'; the full review can be downloaded from the web at http://www.nap.edu/catalog/10534.html. A review published in 2002 recommended that SV 40 should be classified as IARC Group 2, probably carcinogenic to humans, but IARC has not so far carried out an assessment of SV 40[20].

Merkel cell polyomavirus (MCP)

Merkel cell polyomaviruses (MCP) was first isolated in 2008 from Merkel cell carcinoma tissue samples[21]. Merkel cell carcinoma is a rare aggressive neuroendocrine skin neoplasm, most commonly seen in elderly white people[22–25]. The incidence rate is reported to be rising significantly in the US population[26].

It is highly plausible that Merkel cell polyomavirus will eventually be classified as IARC Group 1 but at present it cannot be classified as a proven carcinogen. Known aetiological factors for Merkel cell carcinoma are exposure to ultraviolet light and immunosuppression[27].

Summary

- No polyomavirus has yet been classified as a human carcinogen
- Extensive literature exists hypothesizing that SV 40 is implicated in aetiology of one or more human cancers
- The most persuasive evidence is probably that implicating SV 40 as a cofactor to asbestos in aetiology of mesothelioma
- Merkel cell polyomavirus is a recently described member of the family which has been found in a high proportion of Merkel cell carcinomas

There are no proven instances of polyomaviruses acting as human carcinogens but they are well established as causing tumours in animals, especially in heterologous hosts[1]. There is persuasive evidence that at least one human cancer is caused by a newly discovered polyomavirus[28].

References

1. zur Hausen, H. (2008) Novel human polyomaviruses – Re-emergence of a well known virus family as possible human carcinogens. *International Journal of Cancer*, **123**, 247–250.

2. Neu, U., Stehle, T. & Atwood, W.J. (2009) The Polyomaviridae: Contributions of virus structure to our understanding of virus receptors and infectious entry. *Virology*, **384**, 389–399.

3. Jiang, M., Abend, J.R., Johnson, S.F. & Imperiale, M.J. (2009) The role of polyomaviruses in human disease. *Virology*, **384**, 266–273.

4. Abend, J.R., Jiang, M. & Imperiale, M.J. (2009) BK virus and human cancer: Innocent until proven guilty. *Seminars in Cancer Biology*, **19**, 252–260.

5. IARC Working Group on the Evaluation of Carcinogenic Risks to Humans (2007) Human papillomaviruses. *IARC Monographs on the Evaluation of Carcinogenic Risks to Humans*, **90**, 1–636.

6. Nickeleit, V. & Mihatsch, M.J. (2006) Polyomavirus nephropathy in native kidneys and renal allografts: An update on an escalating threat. *Transplant International*, **19**, 960–973.

7. Epker, J.L., van Biezen, P., van Daele, P.L., van Gelder, T., Vossen, A. & van Saase, J.L. (2009) Progressive multifocal leukoencephalopathy, a review and an extended report of five patients with different immune compromised states. *European Journal of Internal Medicine*, **20**, 261–267.

8. Sweet, B.H. & Hilleman, M.R. (1960) The vacuolating virus, SV 40. *Proceedings of the Society for Experimental Biology and Medicine*, **105**, 420–427.

9. Eddy, B.E., Borman, G.S., Berkeley, W.H. & Young, R.D. (1961) Tumors induced in hamsters by injection of rhesus monkey kidney cell extracts. *Proceedings of the Society for Experimental Biology and Medicine*, **107**, 191–197.

10. Eddy, B.E., Borman, G.S., Grubbs, G.E. & Young, R.D. (1962) Identification of the oncogenic substance in rhesus monkey kidney cell culture as simian virus 40. *Virology*, **17**, 65–75.

11. Gerber, P. & Kirschstein, R.L. (1962) SV40-induced ependymomas in newborn hamsters. I. Virus-tumor relationships. *Virology*, **18**, 582–588.

12. Girardi, A.J., Sweet, B.H., Slotnick, V.B. & Hilleman, M.R. (1962) Development of tumors in hamsters inoculated in the neonatal period with vacuolating virus, SV-40. *Proceedings of the Society for Experimental Biology and Medicine*, **109**, 649–660.

13. Kirschstein, R.L. & Gerber, P. (1962) Ependymomas produced after intracerebral inoculation of SV40 into new-born hamsters. *Nature*, **195**, 299–300.

14. Rabson, A.S., O'Conor, G.T., Kirschstein, R.L. & Branigan, W.J. (1962) Papillary ependymomas produced in Rattus (Mastomys) natalensis inoculated with vacuolating virus (SV40). *Journal of the National Cancer Institute*, **29**, 765–787.

15. Rabson, A.S. & Kirschstein, R.L. (1962) Induction of malignancy in vitro in newborn hamster kidney tissue infected with simian vacuolating virus (SV40). *Proceedings of the Society for Experimental Biology and Medicine*, **111**, 323–328.

16. Huebner, R.J., Chanock, R.M., Rubin, B.A. & Casey, M.J. (1964) Induction by adenovirus type 7 of tumors in hamsters having the antigenic characteristics of SV40 virus. *Proceedings of the National Academy of Sciences of the United States of America*, **52**, 1333–1340.

17. Pipas, J.M. (2009) SV40: Cell transformation and tumorigenesis. *Virology*, **384**, 294–303.

18. Bergsagel, D.J., Finegold, M.J., Butel, J.S., Kupsky, W.J. & Garcea, R.L. (1992) DNA sequences similar to those of simian virus 40 in ependymomas and choroid plexus tumors of childhood. *New England Journal of Medicine*, **326**, 988–993.

19. Stratton, K., Almario, D.A. & McCormick, M.C. (eds) (2002) *Immunization Safety Review: SV40 Contamination of Polio Vaccine and Cancer*. National Academies Press, Washington.

20. Gazdar, A.F., Butel, J.S. & Carbone, M. (2002) SV40 and human tumours: Myth, association or causality? *Nature Reviews Cancer*, **2**, 957–964.

21. Feng, H., Shuda, M., Chang, Y. & Moore, P.S. (2008) Clonal integration of a polyomavirus in human Merkel cell carcinoma. *Science*, **319**, 1096–1100.

22. Heymann, W.R. (2008) Merkel cell carcinoma: Insights into pathogenesis. *Journal of the American Academy of Dermatology*, **59**, 503–504.

23. Becker, J.C., Schrama, D. & Houben, R. (2009) Merkel cell carcinoma. *Cellular and Molecular Life Sciences*, **66**, 1–8.

24. Bichakjian, C.K., Lowe, L., Lao, C.D., *et al.* (2007) Merkel cell carcinoma: Critical review with guidelines for multidisciplinary management. *Cancer*, **110**, 1–12.

25. Pectasides, D., Pectasides, M. & Economopoulos, T. (2006) Merkel cell cancer of the skin. *Annals of Oncology*, **17**, 1489–1495.

26. Hodgson, N.C. (2005) Merkel cell carcinoma: Changing incidence trends. *Journal of Surgical Oncology*, **89**, 1–4.

27. Goessling, W., McKee, P.H. & Mayer, R.J. (2002) Merkel cell carcinoma. *Journal of Clinical Oncology*, **20**, 588–598.

28. Atkin, S.J.L., Griffin, B.E. & Dilworth, S.M. (2009) Polyoma virus and simian virus 40 as cancer models: History and perspectives. *Seminars in Cancer Biology*, **19**, 211–217.

Part II   Bacterial Causes of Cancer

11 *Helicobacter pylori*

Helicobacter pylori is the only bacterium which can colonize the human stomach, and is believed to be the most common chronic bacterial infection globally. Related species are found in many animals, including domestic cats. There is wide geographical and socio-economic variation in incidence; highest incidence is seen in areas and populations of low socio-economic development or status. Infection with *H. pylori* is associated with an increased risk of certain types of stomach cancer[1], including a form of lymphoma. Although the evidence is less clear, infection appears to reduce the risk of oesophageal cancer and of cancer of the gastric cardia.

Infection is becoming less common in the Western world; there is a marked cohort effect (infection rates are lowest amongst the youngest members of the population).

Microbiologists have a special term for those species capable of thriving under one or more physical or chemical extremes such as temperature, pressure, pH or salinity; they are known, aptly, as extremophiles. *H. pylori* is unique since it occupies a niche within the human body which is so hostile as to qualify its flora as extremophile. *Helicobacter* are the only bacteria known to be able to survive the acidity of gastric juices. Survival is achieved, in part, by creating a less hostile micro-environment around the bacterium – an enzyme called urease breaks down urea to yield carbon dioxide and ammonia, thus locally reducing acidity. Urease is only one of *H. pylori*'s stratagems; it can penetrate the stomach wall's protective mucous coating, orientate itself within the layer and migrate down to the epithelial surface where it anchors itself by binding more closely than most bacterial species are capable of doing.

This does not exhaust *H. pylori*'s bag of tricks – it also subverts the immune system – despite triggering both the innate and adaptive immune systems, *H. pylori* still avoids being destroyed[2]. Although the most common cancer associated with *H. pylori* infection is non-cardia gastric cancer there is also an increased risk of lymphoma of the mucosal-associated lymphoid tissue (MALToma) type. This may be directly associated with the chronic inflammation induced by *H. pylori* infection.

Infectious Causes of Cancer, first edition. By Ken Campbell. Published 2011 by John Wiley & Sons Ltd.
© 2011 John Wiley & Sons Ltd.

Where MALToma is detected early it may be cured by eradication of *H. pylori* infection; at later stages the lymphoma will persist even in the absence of *H. pylori*[3].

Helicobacter cannot be classed as a commensal since almost all hosts of *H. pylori* develop chronic gastritis, usually asymptomatic or merely leading to dyspepsia[4]. More severe illness develops in a minority of infected individuals; one might perhaps describe it as an 'accidental pathogen' in those cases where the presence of cofactors leads to development of symptomatic illness. Chronic inflammation has been recognized since the time of Virchow as providing optimal conditions for emergence of cancer[5,6].

The great variability between populations in the proportion of infected individuals who develop ulcers or cancer clearly shows that there must be cofactors required for development of stomach disease. These probably include genetic variation in both host and pathogen, dietary differences and possibly stress; the male:female ratio for gastric cancer ranges between 1.5–4:1 in published studies yet the rate of *H. pylori* is the same in men and women[7]. *H. pylori* infection has been described as 'necessary but not sufficient' for development of gastric cancer[8] or 'a (close to) necessary condition'[9]; this must be qualified as referring specifically to non-cardia gastric cancer, as there is evidence that *H. pylori* infection may reduce the risk of cancer of the gastric cardia[10]. The cardia is that part of the stomach which surrounds the opening of the oesophagus – some epidemiologists have proposed that cancers in this region should be grouped with oesophageal cancer, rather than with other stomach cancers[11]. The term proximal is sometimes used rather than cardia; stomach cancer at other sites is referred to as distal.

It is thought that most, if not all, *H. pylori* infections are acquired very early in life, typically by transmission from mother to infant. There is a very strong cohort effect in rates of infection in the developed world, which is thought to reflect improving hygiene levels leading to a reduced rate of vertical transmission. The infection rate among adults who are seronegative, either *ab-initio* or following eradication therapy, is very low. This is important to proposals that have been made for population-level campaigns to eradicate *H. pylori* using antibiotics[12]; such attempts would be futile unless the risk of re-infection is minimal. Such proposals remain controversial[1], and it has been pointed out that we may well have co-evolved with *H. pylori*[13] and to carry the bacterium may be considered the default state, not to be altered with impunity[14]. It must be made clear that eradication of infection of individual patients who are symptomatic is gold-standard therapy and is wholly uncontroversial[15]; US guidelines consider it controversial whether people deemed high-risk for gastric cancer should have routine diagnosis and treatment of *H. pylori* infection[16].

Historical background

Aeons ago early humans featured in the diet of African big cats; around 200 000 years ago one feline made a poor choice of prey. As well as a meal it acquired a belly-ache that still afflicts many of its descendants now – its victim was infected with the bacterium *H. pylori*[17]; modern cheetahs, lions and tigers still carry a closely related *Helicobacter* species descended from the ones which infected that early cat. As with humans, the big cats are prone to suffer gastritis if they are infected with *Helicobacter* species.

Unfortunately for modern humans, the big cat's hapless victim was clearly not the only early human infected with *H. pylori* – around half the human population now carry *H. pylori* in their stomachs. Minor variations in the genome of *H. pylori* act as molecular milestones tracing the emergence of modern humans from the African Rift Valley. The pattern of infection indicates that about 60 000 years ago, when anatomically modern humans first began to spread across the globe, they were already infected with *H. pylori*[18]. *H. pylori* is the major risk factor for gastric cancer[19], which is second only to lung cancer as a cause of cancer deaths[20]. Given the contribution of *H. pylori* to the aetiology of stomach cancer it is clear that infection associated cancer existed before the emergence of anatomically modern humans. *H. pylori* infection has probably infected a very high proportion of the human population ever since the emergence of anatomically modern humans.

The highest rates of *H. pylori* infection are seen today in the developing world[21], amongst people whose lifestyle and hygiene standards probably reflect those of all humans in prehistoric eras. Blaser has suggested that the modern period is probably the first time in human evolution there have been large numbers of uninfected individuals[14]. Rates of infection are falling within the developed world, but this is not uniform and it is particularly prevalent in the Western world among socially deprived groups including, but not limited to, recent immigrants[22]; in communities where rates of *H. pylori* infection have fallen the rate of gastric cancer has also reduced[23].

The organism now classified as *H. pylori* was first described, over 100 years ago, by Bizzozero[24] – this paper is cited by Marshall in his Nobel lecture[25] as the first report of the presence of spirochaetes in the stomachs of humans and animals. For almost a century the organism was considered to be either a contaminant of samples or an incidental finding; it was believed that no bacterium could colonize the stomach. Although many bacterial species can survive gastric passage the low pH of gastric juice was believed to be too hostile to allow existence of a resident flora. It was not until 1982 that *H. pylori* was cultured from gastric biopsies by pathologist Robin Warren – he reported his success in a letter to the *Lancet* in 1983[26]. Warren's Nobel lecture described how success depended in part on an accident reminiscent of that by which Fleming discovered penicillin. The culture plates from Warren's research study had initially been examined at 48h, as would be normal for clinical samples – as no growth was seen on these plates they were discarded. Over the Easter holiday, the plates were left in the incubator for 5 days and they were found to bear cultures of a new bacterium, not previously described – *H. pylori*[27]. After this, all of Warren's plates were allowed to mature and several more cultures were obtained. Ironically, probably the toughest bacterium in the body is very picky in its culture requirements; *'Cultivation of H. pylori require a microaerophilic atmosphere and complex media'*[28], the accidental extended incubation allowed just such conditions to arise in the culture medium.

In 1984 Warren published a joint paper with gastroenterologist Barry Marshall on the association between *H. pylori* infection and peptic ulceration[29]. Based on its morphology Warren and Marshall initially classified the organism as *Campylobacter pylori* but it was re-classified to the genus *Helicobacter*[30]. Within a decade of Warren's initial letter the evidence linking *H. pylori* to gastric cancer was sufficiently persuasive for International Agency for Research on Cancer (IARC) to classify it as a Group 1 carcinogen – 'Infection with *H. pylori* is *carcinogenic to humans*'[31]. It has been suggested that Napoleon Bonaparte's most probable cause of death was gastric cancer triggered by *H. pylori* infection[32].

Microbiology of Helicobacter pylori

H. pylori is a Gram-negative spiral bacterium about 0.5 μm × 3.0 μm, which is the only organism known to colonize the stomach. Several distinct strains of *H. pylori* exist with differing propensities to cause disease. A key determinant of pathogenicity appears to be the presence or absence of a gene called *cagA*, which codes for a protein called CagA (cytotoxin-associated antigen).

It has a number of adaptations to facilitate survival in the hostile environment of the gastric interior – it is the only organism which can survive the very low pH of gastric juice, far more acidic than other microorganisms can endure.

On first entering the stomach *H. pylori* creates a less hostile micro-environment by using the enzyme urease to break down urea, yielding ammonia and carbon dioxide, both of which act locally to raise the pH to a more tolerable level. *H. pylori* has the ability not only to penetrate the mucous lining the stomach but to orientate itself within the mucous layer and migrate to the region of lowest acidity – adjacent to the gastric epithelium.

Once in contact with the epithelial layer, *H. pylori* form unusually tight bonds with the epithelial cell membrane, allowing 'injection' of bacterial proteins into the cytosol. These bacterial proteins include cytotoxicity-associated antigen (CagA), vacuolating cytotoxin (VacA) and neutrophil-activating protein (NapA) – they are known collectively as virulence factors[28]; expression of the *CagA* gene in particular is thought to significantly influence the risk of developing stomach cancer[33]. Different levels of expression of *CagA* may be a factor in the highly variable correlation between levels of *H. pylori* infection and incidence of related gastric malignancies.

The *CagA* gene is found in a region of the genome called the *cag* pathogenicity-associated island (*cag*PAI); *CagA* is the last gene in the *cag*PAI, which also codes for the proteins of the type IV secretion system by which *H. pylori* inserts the CagA protein. Pathogenicity associated islands are segments of genome which are closely linked and are the best understood example of a general phenomenon known as genetic islands. PAI are associated with the presence of virulence genes and are typically present in pathogens but absent in benign relatives. An excellent review of pathogenicity-associated islands and their role in bacterial virulence is available as free-full text on the web[34].

Associated malignancies

Stomach cancer was known to Hippocrates and Galen; the first clear description was given in the fifteenth century by the Venetian Antonio Benivioni[35]. In the eighteenth century Virchow, the 'father of pathology' described it as the commonest cancer in Germany; he was, of course, writing before the epidemic of tobacco-induced lung cancer. It is now the second commonest cancer in the world, and the fourth commonest in Europe[36]. There are striking variations in the geographic incidence of gastric cancer in the Western world, which may relate both to variations in *H. pylori* infection (rates and strains involved) and to cofactor prevalence[37]. There has been a steady worldwide decline in gastric cancer rates over the last few decades; although the causes of this are not fully understood they are likely to include improved diet and decreased prevalence of *H. pylori* infection[38]. It is highly probably that there have been variations in incidence over a longer historical scale resulting from similar variations in risk factor exposure. It is generally agreed that *H. pylori* infection is associated with an increased risk of non-cardia gastric cancer[39]; whether it affects the risk of cancer of the gastric cardia is more controversial[40].

For some time it was reported that the level of gastric cancer was low in certain areas of Africa, despite high *H. pylori* endemicity[41]. This has been referred to as the 'African enigma' and many potential explanations have been offered[42,43]. A systematic review of prospective endoscopic studies of African populations concluded that the African enigma does not exist; '*The myth resulted from reliance on anecdotal data and selection bias in populations with extremely limited access to health care and a relatively short life expectancy*'[44]. This review has, in turn, been challenged as not explaining discrepancies between African populations with comparable access to healthcare[45]. There is also an 'Asian paradox', referring to the lack of correlation between *H. pylori* infection rates and gastric cancer incidence in some Asian populations[46].

MALToma (Mucosal-associated Lymphoid Tissue lymphoma) is an uncommon form of non-Hodgkin lymphoma which is strongly associated with *H. pylori* infection – early stage lymphoma can be eradicated by clearing the infection with antimicrobial therapy. Normal gastric mucosa contains no lymphoid tissue[47]; as the only gastric pathogen, *H. pylori* is the most common factor inducing migration of lymphocytes into the mucosa. More advanced stages are no longer dependent on the stimulus provided by the presence of *H. pylori*; additional genetic changes allow them to flourish in the absence of the bacterium. MALToma was first described in 1983 by Peter Isaacson[48]. The association between *H. pylori* and MALToma was reported in 1991[49], by Isaacson's team; within 2 years they had demonstrated, in a small study, that eradication of *H. pylori* infection was sufficient to induce clearance of early gastric MALToma[50].

Other malignancies

In mice the related species, *H. hepaticus*, has been found to cause hepatitis and HCC; evidence in humans is equivocal, but would seem to justify further studies[51].

There have been reports of an apparently causal link between *H. pylori* and pancreatic cancer[52,53]. A case report of gastric Burkitt lymphoma resolving after *H. pylori* eradication suggests a possible causal association but cannot be regarded as conclusive evidence[54].

It has been proposed, although it is not universally accepted, that *H. pylori* infection reduces the incidence of gastro-oesophageal reflux disorder (GERD), and thus the risk of oesophageal cancer[55], and possibly of proximal gastric cancers[10]. If this is true it would bolster the argument against routine eradication of *H. pylori* in populations with a low incidence of stomach cancer. In areas with high rates of stomach cancer, the benefit from population-level eradication programmes clearly outweighs any potential harm from increased oesophageal cancer[56]; the rationale for test and treat programmes in developed world populations is much less obvious[57]. In the developed world the rate of decline in *H. pylori* infection in succeeding generations is so striking that the debate on eradication may be purely academic; most people over 60 in Britain are infected with *H. pylori*, compared with only 10%–20% of children[15]. It is thought that there may be multiple causes for this including improved hygiene, smaller families and widespread use of antibiotics during childhood[58].

Cofactors

Several cofactors have been reported to increase the risk of gastric cancer; it is probable that, for the most part, these exert their effect by provoking inflammation. In the case of gastric MALToma, there is less evidence of a role for cofactors.

Proximal gastric cancers

There is strong evidence that bacterial genetic variation influences the risk of a particular infection progressing via gastritis to ulceration and, potentially, malignant transformation; it is also believed that host genetic variation may influence whether infection is harmless or pathogenic[59]. Environmental exposures may also be significant for gastric cancer; particularly diet, smoking and, possibly, betel quid chewing[60]. The IARC monograph on betel quid chewing and stomach cancer cites a single positive paper[61] but rejects this on the basis that the link disappears when corrected for smoking and drinking; a paper published after the monograph reports a significant increased risk associated with areca-consumption (areca nut is a component of betel quids)[62]. Salt has been shown to be a specific dietary risk factor, possibly acting by regulating *CagA* gene expression in *H. pylori*[63]; in Mizoram in India, local dietary peculiarities are thought to explain the high rate of gastric cancer compared to neighbouring areas[64].

Prevention

There are three major determinants of whether *H. pylori* infection is pathogenic or not; the first of these is heterogeneity of the bacterial genome, the second is heterogeneity of host susceptibility, and the last is the presence or absence of cofactors, which may be preventive or increase risk[65].

Although there is nothing that can be done directly about the genetics of the organism, it has been suggested that it may be feasible to take this into account in deciding which populations are likely to benefit from eradication programs[66]. Heterogeneity of host susceptibility may be relevant at national level in determining the need for eradication; Japanese *Helicobacter* researchers are reported to be petitioning their government to eradicate *H. pylori* in the Japanese population[67]. The WHO has taken a rather different tack on gastric cancer prevention; given the widespread consensus that dietary risk factors contribute to the geographical heterogeneity of gastric cancer they prefer to promote healthy diet and exercise, on the basis that this will also reduce the risk of other forms of cancer[68]. In developed nations it is arguable that the benefits from addressing cofactors such as smoking and poor diet would offer additional substantial health benefits. Given the striking decline in *H. pylori* infection levels and gastric cancer incidence and the potential for induction of microbial resistance a rational policy for the UK would be to confine test-and-treat to high-risk groups.

Summary

- *H. pylori* is the only bacterium which can colonize the human stomach
  - It is believed to be the most common chronic bacterial infection globally
  - There are related species in many animals, including domestic cats
  - There is wide geographical and socio-economic variation in incidence; highest incidence is seen in areas and populations of low socio-economic development or status
- Infection is associated with an increased risk of certain types of stomach cancer, including a form of lymphoma
- Although the evidence is less clear, infection appears to reduce the risk of oesophageal cancer and of cancer of the gastric cardia
- Infection is becoming less common in the Western world, with a marked cohort effect

H. pylori is perhaps the most widespread human bacterial infection and yet, because it inhabits such a hostile anatomical niche, its very existence went unsuspected until recently. It is believed to have co-evolved with humans and it has been suggested that humans are adapted to coexist with the organism and population-level eradication programmes may be harmful by increasing the incidence of certain malignant and non-malignant conditions.

At an individual level, it has been shown that eradication of *H. pylori* infection can reverse early stage gastric MALToma and will reduce the risk of recurrence following treatment for *H. pylori* related gastric cancer. The rate of acquisition of *H. pylori* during adult life is very low, so the benefit of eradication is not compromised by re-infection.

References

1. Kim, W. & Moss, S.F. (2008) The role of *Helicobacter pylori* in the pathogenesis of gastric malignancies. *Oncology Review*, **2**, 131–140.

2. Chui, S.Y., Clay, T.M., Lyerly, H.K. & Morse, M.A. (2005) The development of therapeutic and preventive vaccines for gastric cancer and *Helicobacter pylori*. *Cancer Epidemiology, Biomarkers and Prevention*, **14**, 1883–1889.

3. Isaacson, P.G. (2005) Update on MALT lymphomas. *Best Practice and Research Clinical Haematology*, **18**, 57–68.

4. Dooley, C.P., Cohen, H., Fitzgibbons, P.L., *et al.* (1989) Prevalence of *Helicobacter pylori* infection and histologic gastritis in asymptomatic persons. *New England Journal of Medicine*, **321**, 1562–1566.

5. Bertout, J. & Thomas-Tikhonenko, A. (2006) Infection & neoplastic growth 101: The required reading for microbial pathogens aspiring to cause cancer. *Cancer Treatment and Research*, **130**, 167–197.

6. Dalgleish, A.G. & O'Byrne, K. (2006) Inflammation and cancer: The role of the immune response and angiogenesis. *Cancer Treatment and Research*, **130**, 1–38.

7. Khanna, A.K., Seth, P., Nath, G., Dixit, V.K. & Kumar, M. (2002) Correlation of *Helicobacter pylori* and gastric carcinoma. *Journal of Postgraduate Medicine*, **48**, 27–28.

8. Graham, D.Y. & Shiotani, A. (2005) The time to eradicate gastric cancer is now. *Gut*, **54**, 735–738.

9. Brenner, H., Arndt, V., Stegmaier, C., Ziegler, H. & Rothenbacher, D. (2004) Is *Helicobacter pylori* infection a necessary condition for noncardia gastric cancer? *American Journal of Epidemiology*, **159**, 252–258.

10. Kamangar, F., Dawsey, S.M., Blaser, M.J., *et al.* (2006) Opposing risks of gastric cardia and noncardia gastric adeonocarcinoma associated with *Helicobacter pylori* seropositivity. *Journal of the National Cancer Institute*, **98**, 1445–1452.

11. Driessen, A., Van Raemdonck, D., De Leyn, P., *et al.* (2003) Are carcinomas of the cardia oesophageal or gastric adenocarcinomas? *European Journal of Cancer*, **39**, 2487–2494.

12. Graham, D.Y. (1997) The only good *Helicobacter pylori* is a dead *Helicobacter pylori*. *Lancet*, **350**, 70–71.

13. Blaser, M.J. (2006) Who are we? Indigenous microbes and the ecology of human diseases. *EMBO Reports*, **7**, 956–960.

14. Blaser, M.J. (1999) Hypothesis: The changing relationships of *Helicobacter pylori* and humans: Implications for health and disease. *Journal of Infectious Disease*, **179**, 1523–1530.

15. Fuccio, L., Laterza, L., Zagari, R.M., Cennamo, V., Grilli, D. & Bazzoli, F. (2008) Treatment of *Helicobacter pylori* infection. *BMJ*, **337**, 746–750.

16. Chey, W.D. & Wong, B.C. (2007) American college of gastroenterology guideline on the management of *Helicobacter pylori* infection. *American Journal of Gastroenterology*, 102, 1808–1825.

17. Eppinger, M., Baar, C., Linz, B., *et al.* (2006) Who ate whom? Adaptive *Helicobacter* genomic changes that accompanied a host jump from early humans to large felines. *PLoS Genetics*, **2**, 1097–1110.

18. Linz, B., Balloux, F., Moodley, Y., *et al.* (2007) An African origin for the intimate association between humans and *Helicobacter pylori*. *Nature*, **445** (7130), 915–918.

19. Pinto-Santini, D. & Salama, N.R. (2005) The biology of *Helicobacter pylori* infection, a major risk factor for gastric adenocarcinoma. *Cancer Epidemiology, Biomarkers and Prevention*, **14**, 1853–1858.

20. Hunt, R.H. (2004) Will eradication of *Helicobacter pylori* infection influence the risk of gastric cancer? *American Journal of Medicine*, **117** (Suppl. 5A), 86S–91S.

21. Marshall, B.J. & Windsor, H.M. (2005) The relation of *Helicobacter pylori* to gastric adenocarcinoma and lymphoma: Pathophysiology, epidemiology, screening, clinical presentation, treatment, and prevention. *Medical Clinics of North America*, **89**, 313–44, viii.

22. Fennerty, M.B. (2005) *Helicobacter pylori*: Why it still matters in 2005. *Cleveland Clinical Journal of Medicine*, 72 (Suppl. 2), S1–S7; discussion S14–S21.

23. Parsonnet, J., Blaser, M.J., Perez-Perez, G.I., Hargrett-Bean, N. & Tauxe, R.V. (1992) Symptoms and risk factors of *Helicobacter pylori* infection in a cohort of epidemiologists. *Gastroenterology*, **102**, 42–46.

24. Bizzozero, G. (1892) Sulle ghiandole tubulari del tube gastroenterico e sui rapporti dell'ero coll epithelo de rivestimento della mucosa. *Atti Della Reale Academia Delle Scienze Di Torino*, **28**, 233–251.

25. Marshall, B. (2006) *Helicobacter* connections. *ChemMedChem*, **1**, 783–802.

26. Warren, J.R. (1983) Unidentified curved bacilli on gastric epithelium in active chronic gastritis. *Lancet*, **1**, 1273–1275.

27. Warren, J.R. (2006) *Helicobacter* – the ease and difficulty of a new discovery. *Le Prix Nobel.* *Stockholm* The Nobel Foundation 292–305.

28. Pinto-Santini, D. & Salama, N.R. (2005) The biology of *Helicobacter pylori* infection, a major risk factor for gastric adenocarcinoma. *Cancer Epidemiology, Biomarkers and Prevention*, **14**, 1853–1858.

29. Marshall, B.J. & Warren, J.R. (1984) Unidentified curved bacilli in the stomach of patients with gastritis and peptic ulceration. *Lancet*, **1**, 1311–1315.

30. Goodwin, C.S., Armstrong, J.A., Chilvers, T., *et al.* (1989) Transfer of *Campylobacter pylori* and *C. mustelae* to *Helicobacter* gen. nov. as *Helicobacter pylori* comb. nov. and *H. mustelae* com. nov., respectively. *International Journal of Systematic Bacteriology*, **39**, 397–405.

31. IARC (1994) Infection with *Helicobacter pylori*. In: *Schistosomes, Liver Flukes and Helicobacter pylori* (eds IARC), pp. 177–240. International Agency for Research on Cancer, Lyon.

32. Lugli, A., Zlobec, I., Singer, G., Kopp, L.A., Terracciano, L.M. & Genta, R.M. (2007) Napoleon Bonaparte's gastric cancer: A clinicopathologic approach to staging, pathogenesis, and etiology. *Nature Clinical Practice Gastroenterology and Hepatology*, **4**, 52–57.

33. Ahmed, N. & Sechi, L.A. (2005) *Helicobacter pylori* and gastroduodenal pathology: New threats of the old friend. *Annals of Clinical Microbiology and Antimicrobials*, **4** (1), 1.

34. Schmidt, H. & Hensel, M. (2004) Pathogenicity islands in bacterial pathogenesis. *Clinical Microbiology Review*, **17**, 14–56.

35. Greaves, M.F. (2000) Soot, civilization, and neuroses. *Cancer. The Evolutionary Legacy*, pp. 13–19. Oxford University Press, Oxford.

36. Shang, J. & Pena, A.S. (2005) Multidisciplinary approach to understand the pathogenesis of gastric cancer. *World Journal of Gastroenterology*, **11**, 4131–4139.

37. Liu, Y., Ponsioen, C.I., Xiao, S.D., Tytgat, G.N. & ten Kate, F.J. (2005) Geographic pathology of *Helicobacter pylori* gastritis. *Helicobacter*, **10**, 107–113.

38. Plummer, M., Franceschi, S. & Munoz, N. (2004) Epidemiology of gastric cancer. *IARC Science Publication*, **157**, 311–326.

39. Gurjeet, K., Subathra, S. & Bhupinder, S. (2004) Differences in the pattern of gastric carcinoma between north-eastern and north-western peninsular Malaysia: A reflection of *Helicobacter pylori* prevalence. *Medical Journal of Malaysia*, **59**, 560–561.

40. Kato, M., Asaka, M., Shimizu, Y., Nobuta, A., Takeda, H. & Sugiyama, T. (2004) Relationship between *Helicobacter pylori* infection and the prevalence, site and histological type of gastric cancer. *Alimentary Pharmacology and Therapeutics*, **20** (Suppl. 1), 85–89.

41. Holcombe, C. (1992) *Helicobacter pylori*: The African enigma. *Gut*, **33**, 429–431.

42. Lunet, N. & Barros, H. (2003) *Helicobacter pylori* infection and gastric cancer: Facing the enigmas. *International Journal of Cancer*, **106**, 953–960.

43. Bravo, L.E., van Doom, L.J., Realpe, J.L. & Correa, P. (2002) Virulence-associated genotypes of *Helicobacter pylori*: Do they explain the African enigma? *American Journal of Gastroenterology*, **97**, 2839–2842.

44. Agha, A. & Graham, D.Y. (2005) Evidence-based examination of the African enigma in relation to *Helicobacter pylori* infection. *Scandinavian Journal of Gastroenterology*, **40**, 523–529.

45. Mbulaiteye, S.M., Gold, B.D., Pfeiffer, R.M., *et al.* (2006) *H. pylori*-infection and antibody immune response in a rural Tanzanian population. *Infectious Agents and Cancer*, **1**, 3.

46. Matsukura, N., Yamada, S., Kato, S., *et al.* (2003) Genetic differences in interleukin-1 betapolymorphisms among four Asian populations: An analysis of the Asian paradox between *H. pylori* infection and gastric cancer incidence. *Journal of Experimental and Clinical Cancer Research*, **22**, 47–55.

47. Du, M.Q. & Isaccson, P.G. (2002) Gastric MALT lymphoma: From aetiology to treatment. *Lancet Oncology*, **3**, 97–104.

48. Isaacson, P.G. & Wright, D.H. (1983) Malignant lymphoma of mucosa-associated lymphoid tissue. A distinctive type of B cell lymphoma. *Cancer*, **52**, 1410–1416.

49. Wotherspoon, A.C., Ortiz-Hidalgo, C., Falzon, M.R. & Isaacson, P.G. (1991) *Helicobacter pylori*-associated gastritis and primary B-cell gastric lymphoma. *Lancet*, **338**, 1175–1176.

50. Wotherspoon, A.C., Doglioni, C., Diss, T.C., *et al.* (1993) Regression of primary low-grade B-cell gastric lymphoma of mucosa-associated lymphoid tissue type after eradication of *Helicobacter pylori*. *Lancet*, **342**, 575–577.

51. Pellicano, R., Menard, A., Rizzetto, M. & Megraud, F. (2008) *Helicobacter* species and liver diseases: Association or causation? *Lancet Infectious Disease*, **8**, 254–260.

52. Nilsson, H.O., Stenram, U., Ihse, I. & Wadstrom, T. (2006) *Helicobacter* species ribosomal DNA in the pancreas, stomach and duodenum of pancreatic cancer patients. *World Journal of Gastroenterology*, **12**, 3038–3043.

53. Luo, J., Nordenvall, C., Nyren, O., Adami, H.O., Permert, J. & Ye, W. (2007) The risk of pancreatic cancer in patients with gastric or duodenal ulcer disease. *International Journal of Cancer*, **120**, 368–372.

54. Baumgaernter, I., Copie-Bergman, C., Levy, M., *et al.* (2009) Complete remission of gastric Burkitt's lymphoma after eradication of *Helicobacter pylori*. *World Journal of Gastroenterology*, **15**, 5746–5750.

55. Anderson, L.A., Murphy, S.J., Johnston, B.T., *et al.* (2008) Relationship between *Helicobacter pylori* infection and gastric atrophy and the stages of the oesophageal inflammation, metaplasia, adenocarcinoma sequence: Results from the FINBAR case-control study. *Gut*, **57**, 734–739.

56. Tsuji, S., Tsujii, M., Murata, H., *et al.* (2006) *Helicobacter pylori* eradication to prevent gastric cancer: underlying molecular and cellular mechanisms. *World Journal of Gastroenterology*, **12**, 1671–1680.

57. Prinz, C., Schwendy, S. & Voland, P. (2006) *H. pylori* and gastric cancer: Shifting the global burden. *World Journal of Gastroenterology*, **12**, 5458–5464.

58. Roder, D.M. (2002) The epidemiology of gastric cancer. *Gastric Cancer*, **5** (Suppl. 1), 5–11.

59. Akhter, Y., Ahmed, I., Devi, S.M. & Ahmed, N. (2007) The co-evolved *Helicobacter pylori* and gastric cancer: Trinity of bacterial virulence, host susceptibility and lifestyle. *Infectious Agents and Cancer*, **2**, 2.

60. Machida-Montani, A., Sasazuki, S., Inoue, M., *et al.* (2004) Association of *Helicobacter pylori* infection and environmental factors in non-cardia gastric cancer in Japan. *Gastric Cancer*, **7**, 46–53.

61. Gajalakshmi, V. & Shanta, V. (1996) Lifestyle and risk of stomach cancer: A hospital-based case-control study. *International Journal of Epidemiology*, **25**, 1146–1153.

62. Wu, M.T., Chen, M.C. & Wu, D.C. (2004) Influences of lifestyle habits and p53 codon 72 and p21 codon 31 polymorphisms on gastric cancer risk in Taiwan. *Cancer Letters*, **205**, 61–68.

63. Loh, J.T., Torres, V.J. & Cover, T.L. (2007) Regulation of *Helicobacter pylori* cagA expression in response to salt. *Cancer Research*, **67**, 4709–4715.

64. Phukan, R.K., Narain, K., Zomawia, E., Hazarika, N.C. & Mahanta, J. (2006) Dietary habits and stomach cancer in Mizoram, India. *Journal of Gastroenterology*, **41**, 418–424.

65. Ando, T., Goto, Y., Ishiguro, K., *et al.* (2007) The interaction of host genetic factors and *Helicobacter pylori* infection. *Inflammopharmacology*, **15**, 10–14.

66. Yamaoka, Y., Kato, M. & Asaka, M. (2008) Geographic differences in gastric cancer incidence can be explained by differences between *Helicobacter pylori* strains. *Internal Medicine*, **47**, 1077–1083.

67. Talley, N.J. (2008) Is it time to screen and treat *H. pylori* to prevent gastric cancer? *Lancet*, **372**, 350–352.

68. McNeil, C. (2008) *Helicobacter pylori*: Good side complicates efforts to combat bad side. *Journal of National Cancer Institute*, **100**, 1748–1750.

Part III   Parasitic Causes of Cancer

12 Schistosome species

Schistosoma are multicellular parasites with complex lifestyles; their definitive hosts are mammals, including man, while the intermediate hosts are freshwater snails. Transmission is by contact with contaminated water, with larval stages penetrating through intact skin. Infection with one species – *Schistosoma haematobium* – is considered by International Agency for Research on Cancer (IARC) to be a definite human carcinogen. Two other species – *S. japonicum* and *S. mansoni* – have been linked with cancer but are not classed by IARC as carcinogens; *S. japonicum* is classed as possibly carcinogenic and *S. mansoni* is not classifiable. Schistosome infections cannot be acquired or transmitted in the UK because their intermediate hosts are not present.

The organism[1]

Only *S. haematobium* will be discussed in detail here. Apart from their geographical distribution and their intermediate hosts, the species are more similar than different. *S. haematobium* is found in Africa and the Middle East, while *S. japonicum* and *S. mansoni* are found in Japan and the Far East. The illness caused by schistosome infestation may be referred to as bilharzia, in tribute to Theodor Bilharz, who described the parasite in 1852. Recognizable descriptions of the illness can be found in the oldest Egyptian records; as long ago as 3000 BC bilharzia was recognized as being caused by a *'worm in the belly'*[2].

Schistosomes, which are sometimes called blood flukes, are trematode worms. The adult parasites are white or greyish worms which vary between 7 and 20 mm long. They have a cylindrical body, and are found anchored within the venous plexus of the urinary bladder (*S. haematobium*) or the mesentery (other schistosome species). Unlike other trematodes, they have separate sexes; the male's body forms a long groove called the gynaecophoric channel and, once they have paired, the female remains lodged in this groove[3] (see Figure 12.1). The female worm can elect to transfer to a more genetically suitable male – divorce in the schistosome world

Infectious Causes of Cancer, first edition. By Ken Campbell. Published 2011 by John Wiley & Sons Ltd.
© 2011 John Wiley & Sons Ltd.

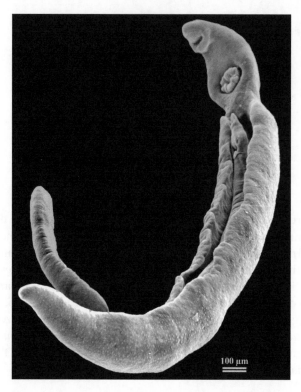

Figure 12.1 A schistosome pair, with the thin female located in the male gynaecophorical canal. (From Beltran *et al.*[3])

is exclusively a female option[3]. They feed on blood and on globins within the plasma, regurgitating indigestible remnants back into the bloodstream. Once lodged in place, the adults live for an average of 3–5 years, although survival for three decades has been recorded.

The female lays large numbers of eggs directly into the bloodstream. The ovum can penetrate the wall of the bladder or gut and enter the lumen. On being excreted in urine or faeces the ovum is viable for up to a week. On contact with fresh water, the ovum releases a larval form called a miracidium, which will seek out and penetrate an intermediate host, a freshwater snail; different schistosome species have different intermediate host species, which is a key factor in limiting their range.

Within a snail, the miracidium will multiply and mature into large numbers of cercarial larvae. The cercarial larvae can live for up to 3 days in fresh water seeking the skin of a host. Even a brief immersion in contaminated water risks infection; a single snail, infected by a single miracidium can release thousands of cercariae a day for many weeks. On contact with a suitable host, cercariae penetrate the intact skin and travel in the circulation to the lung. From the lung they migrate to the liver; within the portal vein they mature, find and permanently bond to a mate and migrate to their final destination.

Initial penetration of cercariae may trigger an urticarial rash; this may be triggered by animal species resident in temperate regions although these cannot establish infection in humans. This is known as 'swimmer's itch' – it is clinically important because anyone who has experienced such symptoms after bathing in areas where *S. haematobium*, *S. japonicum* or *S. mansoni* are endemic must be referred to specialist tropical medicine unit for assessment. There is also an acute presentation of schistosomiasis known as *katayama*; this is characterized by '*nocturnal fever, cough, myalgia, headache, and abdominal tenderness*'[4]. *S. haematobium infection* leads to haematuria; this association is so consistent that this has been validated as a surrogate for urine microscopy in screening programmes in endemic areas[5]. Fortunately, the condition is readily eradicated with a brief course of treatment with praziquantel; there is however anxiety that use of praziquantel prophylactically in eradication programmes in sub-Saharan Africa may lead to drug resistance[6–8].

It should be stressed in advice to travellers to endemic areas that even very brief exposure of unprotected skin to contaminated fresh water is enough for infection to be established[9]. Diagnosis of established infection is based on the discovery of schistosome ova in the urine (*S. haematobium*) or the faeces (other *Schistosome* spp.)[10].

Chronic pathology in schistosome infection, including *S. haematobium*, is not caused by the adult worms but by parasite eggs which become trapped in the tissues or in the vessels, instead of being released in urine or faeces to perpetuate their life cycle. The eggs achieve release by secreting proteolytic enzymes, when the egg is trapped these trigger local inflammatory reactions leading to granuloma formation and to calcification. Schistosome ova have been discovered in Egyptian mummies over 3000 years old[11,12].

Associated malignancies

Chronic urinary schistosomiasis is epidemiologically linked with squamous bladder cancer. The link is sufficiently strong for the IARC to classify infection with *S. haematobium* as Group I – definitely a carcinogen in humans.

Bladder cancer[13,14]

Globally, the most common histological type of bladder cancer is urothelial cancer (also known as transitional cell carcinoma, TCC); this affects the specialized epithelium lining almost the whole of the urinary tract; this includes the renal pelvis, the ureters, the bladder and the proximal part of the urethra. This is known as *urothelium* or *transitional epithelium*; it is specialized both to cope with the marked changes in bladder volume and with prolonged exposure to carcinogens excreted in urine[15]. The principal risk factors for urothelial cancer are cigarette smoking and industrial carcinogen exposure[16].

The type most commonly seen in association with *S. haematobium* infection is squamous cell carcinoma of the bladder[17]. Squamous epithelium does not normally occur in the bladder; it arises in the course of an inflammatory response. This process – replacement of one type of cell by another type not normally found in the anatomical site within a tissue is called metaplasia[18]. Replacement of transitional epithelium with squamous epithelium is thus called *squamous metaplasia*.

In the developed world squamous cell carcinoma (SCC) is uncommon with up to 99% of all bladder cancer being of the TCC type. In Egypt, until recently, the ratio was reversed, with up to three-quarters of all bladder cancer being squamous cell type and schistosomiasis-associated bladder cancer (SABC) being the commonest cancer in men; male bladder cancer mortality was the highest in the world[19,20].

The mechanism of SABC was once thought to be principally, if not solely, focal inflammation leading to hyperplasia and thus predisposing to cancer. It is now thought to be rather more complex with multiple mechanisms[21], including:

■ Inflammatory reactions and elevated cell proliferation[22]
■ Chronic bacteriuria which releases nitrosamines from precursor compounds[2,23]
■ Urinary stasis, increasing absorption of endogenous carcinogens from urine[24]
■ Raised urine β-glucuronidase levels derived from carcinogenic amines released by miracidia and from adult worms[25]

It has recently been reported that *S. haematobium* antigens may directly induce cancer-predisposing changes in normal epithelial cells[26]. The genetic differences between SABC and other bladder cancers are not great, suggesting a common carcinogenic mechanism[27]. This implies that the excess of squamous cell carcinoma occurs because squamous epithelium is only found in the bladder as a result of parasite-induced metaplasia.

The latency between infection and development of cancer may be very long; it is vital to consider the possibility in any person who has spent time in an area where *S. haematobium* is endemic.

Cofactors

The most clearly identified cofactor is cigarette smoking, for squamous cell carcinoma as for transitional cell carcinoma[28]. It is probable that occupational chemical exposures would also increase the risk, but these have not been analysed separately by histological tumour type[29].

Prevention

Endeavours have been made to reduce the disease burden from schistosomal infection – these have variously involved chemotherapy-based eradication programmes[30], sometimes alongside use of molluscicides to eliminate the intermediate host[31]; this approach has proved very successful in Mauritius[32]. The Egyptian National Cancer Institute has reported a decline in the overall incidence of bladder cancer and a reversal from SCC being most common to TCC being more frequent, and that this follows considerable success in controlling bilharzia in rural populations in Egypt[33]. In 2010 an updated strategy was proposed which would incorporate primary health providers to overcome persistent foci of infection[34].

In 1997 the World Health Organization declared development of an anti-schistosomal vaccine as a priority target[35]; the unfortunate lack of progress on this front can be seen from a 2009 *New England Journal of Medicine* editorial which indicates the components of an integrated control strategy as '*a combination of drug treatment, water management, snail control (through habitat modification, irrigation changes, and the use of molluscicidal sprays), and the control or treatment of sewage*'[36].

Summary

- Schistosomes are multicellular parasites with complex lifestyles
  - Definitive hosts are mammals, including man
  - Intermediate hosts are freshwater snails
- Transmission is by contact with contaminated water
  - The larval stage is capable of penetrating intact skin
- Infection with one species – S. haematobium – is considered by IARC to be a definite human carcinogen
  - Two other species – S. japonicum and S. mansoni have been linked with cancer but are not classed by IARC as carcinogens
    - S. japonicum is classed as possibly carcinogenic
    - S. mansoni is not classifiable
- Schistosome infections cannot be acquired or transmitted in the UK because their intermediate hosts are not present

The intermediate hosts for *Schistosoma* species are not found in the UK, thus ruling out transmission or acquisition of the infection. The number of cases annually reported is low, but not low enough to justify complacency. It is important to remember that a full clinical history should always include a travel history. It is also vital that healthcare professionals should be able to offer accurate advice on the measures needed to avoid infection when travelling to endemic areas. In cases presenting in the UK the most common location of infection has been sub-Saharan Africa, particularly around Lake Malawi. Once diagnosed schistosome infection can usually be eradicated with a short course of praziquantel.

References

1. Gryseels, B., Polman, K., Clerinx, J. & Kestens, L. (2006) Human schistosomiasis. *Lancet*, **368**, 1106–1118.
2. Hicks, R.M. (1983) The canopic worm: Role of bilharziasis in the aetiology of human bladder cancer. *Journal of the Royal Society of Medicine*, **76**, 16–22.

3. Beltran, S., Cezilly, F. & Boissier, J. (2008) Genetic dissimilarity between mates, but not male heterozygosity, influences divorce in schistosomes. *PLoS One*, **3**, e3328.

4. Ross, A.G., Vickers, D., Olds, G.R., Shah, S.M. & McManus, D.P. (2007) Katayama syndrome. *The Lancet Infectious Diseases*, **7**, 218–224.

5. Nduka, F.O. & Nwosu, E.C. (2008) Validation of the World Health Organization's rapid assessment method for urinary schistosomiasis in southeastern Nigeria. *Journal of Parasitology*, **94**, 533–536.

6. Doenhoff, M.J., Hagan, P., Cioli, D., *et al.* (2009) Praziquantel: Its use in control of schistosomiasis in sub-Saharan Africa and current research needs. *Parasitology*, **136**(13), 1825–1835.

7. Loukas, A. & Bethony, J.M. (2008) New drugs for an ancient parasite. *Nature Medicine*, **14**, 365–367.

8. Sayed, A.A., Simeonov, A., Thomas, C.J., Inglese, J., Austin, C.P. & Williams, D.L. (2008) Identification of oxadiazoles as new drug leads for the control of schistosomiasis. *Nature Medicine*, **14**, 407–412.

9. Salvana, E.M. & King, C.H. (2008) Schistosomiasis in travelers and immigrants. *Current Infectious Disease Reports*, **10**, 42–49.

10. Ross, A.G., Bartley, P.B., Sleigh, A.C., *et al.* (2002) Schistosomiasis. *New England Journal of Medicine*, **346**, 1212–1220.

11. Ibrahim, A.S. & Khaled, H.M. (2006) Urinary bladder cancer. In: *Cancer Incidence in Four Member Countries (Cyprus, Egypt, Israel and Jordan) of the Middle East Cancer Consortium (MECC) Compared with US SEER* (eds L.S. Freedman, B.K. Edwards, L.A.G. Ries & J.L. Young), pp. 97–110. National Cancer Institute, Bethesda, Maryland.

12. Ruffer, M.A. (1910) Note on the presence of "Bilharzia haematobia" in Egyptian mummies of the twentieth dynasty (1250–1000 B.C.). *BMJ*, **1**, 16.

13. Boyle, P. & Levin, B. (2008) Bladder cancer. In: *World Cancer Report 2008* (eds P. Boyle & B. Levin), pp. 444–449. International Agency for Research on Cancer, Lyon.

14. Eble, J.N., Sauter, G., Epstein, J.I. & Sesterhenn, I.A. (2004) *World Health Organization Classification of Tumours. Pathology and Genetics of Tumours of the Urinary System and Male Genital Organs.* International Agency for Research on Cancer, Lyon.

15. Wheater, P.R., Burkitt, H.G. & Daniels, V.G. (1987) Epithelial tissues. In: *Functional Histology: A Text and Colour Atlas* (eds P.R. Wheater, H.G. Burkitt & V.G. Daniels), pp. 64–78. Churchill Livingstone, Edinburgh.

16. Wu, X.R. (2005) Urothelial tumorigenesis: A tale of divergent pathways. *Nature Reviews Cancer*, **5**, 713–725.

17. IARC (1994) Schistosomes, liver flukes and *Helicobacter pylori*. IARC Working Group on the evaluation of carcinogenic risks to humans. Lyon, 7–14 June 1994. *IARC Monographs on the Evaluation of Carcinogenic Risks to Humans*, **61**, 1–241.

18. Weinberg, R.A. (2007) The nature of cancer. In: *The Biology of Cancer*, pp. 25–56. Garland Science, New York.

19. Elsebai, I. (1977) Parasites in the etiology of cancer – Bilharziasis and bladder cancer. *CA: A Cancer Journal for Clinicians*, **27**, 100–106.

20. Parkin, D.M. (2008) The global burden of urinary bladder cancer. *Scandinavian Journal of Urology and Nephrology*, **42** (Suppl. 218), 12–20.

21. Mostafa, M.H., Sheweita, S.A. & O'Connor, P.J. (1999) Relationship between schistosomiasis and bladder cancer. *Clinical Microbiology Reviews*, **12**, 97–111.

22. Rosin, M.P., Saad el Din Zaki S., Ward, A.J. & Anwar, W.A. (1994) Involvement of inflammatory reactions and elevated cell proliferation in the development of bladder cancer in schistosomiasis patients. *Mutation Research*, **305**, 283–292.

23. Hicks, R.M., Ismail, M.M., Walters, C.L., Beecham, P.T., Rabie, M.F. & El Alamy, M.A. (1982) Association of bacteriuria and urinary nitrosamine formation with Schistosoma haematobium infection in the Qalyub area of Egypt. *Transactions of the Royal Society of Tropical Medicine and Hygiene*, **76**, 519–527.

24. Cheever, A.W. (1978) Schistosomiasis and neoplasia. *Journal of the National Cancer Institute*, **61**, 13–18.

25. Lucas, S.B. (1982) Squamous cell carcinoma of the bladder and schistosomiasis. *East African Medical Journal*, **59**, 345–351.

26. Botelho, M., Ferreira, A.C., Oliveira, M.J., Domingues, A., Machado, J.C. & Costa, J.M. (2009) *Schistosoma haematobium* total antigen induces increased proliferation, migration and invasion, and decreases apoptosis of normal epithelial cells. *International Journal of Parasitology*, **39**(10), 1083–1091.

27. Armengol, G., Eissa, S., Lozano, J.J., *et al.* (2007) Genomic imbalances in schistosoma-associated and non-schistosoma-associated bladder carcinoma. An array comparative genomic hybridization analysis. *Cancer Genetics and Cytogenetics*, **177**, 16–19.

28. Fortuny, J., Kogevinas, M., Chang-Claude, J., *et al.* (1999) Tobacco, occupation and non-transitional-cell carcinoma of the bladder: An international case-control study. *International Journal of Cancer*, **80**, 44–46.

29. Grignon, D.J., El-Bolkainy, M.N., Schmitz-Dräger, B.J., Simon, R. & Tyczynski, J.E. (2004) Tumours of the urinary system – Squamous cell carcinoma In: *World Health Organization Classification of Tumours. Pathology and Genetics of Tumours of the Urinary System and Male Genital Organs* (eds J.N. Eble, G. Sauter, J.I. Epstein & I.A. Sesterhenn), pp. 124–127. International Agency for Research on Cancer, Lyon.

30. King, C.H., Lombardi, G., Lombardi, C., *et al.* (1988) Chemotherapy-based control of schistosomiasis haematobia. I. Metrifonate versus praziquantel in control of intensity and prevalence of infection. *American Journal of Tropical Medicine and Hygiene*, **39**, 295–305.

31. Adewunmi, C.O., Gebremedhin, G., Becker, W., Olurunmola, F.O., Dorfler, G. & Adewunmi, T.A. (1993) Schistosomiasis and intestinal parasites in rural villages in southwest Nigeria: An indication for expanded programme on drug distribution and integrated control programme in Nigeria. *Tropical Medicine and Parasitology*, **44**, 177–180.

32. Dhunputh, J. (1994) Progress in the control of schistosomiasis in Mauritius. *Transactions of the Royal Society of Tropical Medicine and Hygiene*, **88**, 507–509.

33. Gouda, I., Mokhtar, N., Bilal, D., El Bolkainy, T. & El Bolkainy, N.M. (2007) Bilharziasis and bladder cancer: A time trend analysis of 9843 patients. *Journal of the Egyptian National Cancer Institute*, **19**, 158–162.

34. Curtale, F., Mohamed, M.Y. & Youssef, Z.M. (2010) Comprehensive primary health care, a viable strategy for the elimination of schistosomiasis. *Transactions of the Royal Society of Tropical Medicine and Hygiene*, **104**, 70–72.

35. Waine, G.J. & McManus, D.P. (1997) Schistosomiasis vaccine development – The current picture. *Bioessays*, **19**, 435–443.

36. King, C.H. (2009) Toward the elimination of schistosomiasis. *New England Journal of Medicine*, **360**, 106–109.

13 Liver flukes

Liver flukes are multicellular parasites which belong to the trematode family[1]. Two species of liver flukes are classed as carcinogens by International Agency for Research on Cancer (IARC) and for one species the evidence is equivocal.

Opisthorchis viverrini	Group 1 (definite carcinogen)
Clonorchis sinensis	Group 1 (definite carcinogen)
O. viverrini	Group 3 (not classifiable)

Liver fluke infection is associated with cholangiocarcinoma. Liver flukes do not occur naturally and cannot be transmitted in Europe because the intermediate hosts are absent; animal species are found throughout the world, but are not transmissible to humans. The parasites are common throughout South-East Asia and cause serious disease burden.

Although liver flukes do not occur in Europe, South-East Asia has a very large population of chronically infected individuals. It is possible that European healthcare practitioners may encounter patients who have acquired the infection in endemic areas; there are reports of this from the United States[2]. There have also been isolated reports of infection resulting from the consumption of imported raw fish dishes[3]. Latency between infection and malignancy is typically decades long. Infection occurs only by ingestion of raw or poorly cooked fish containing intermediate forms of the parasite.

Organisms[4]

C. sinensis and O. viverrini

There are many common features to the liver flukes *C. sinensis* and *O. viverrini*, so they will be discussed together; significant differences will be highlighted.

Infectious Causes of Cancer, first edition. By Ken Campbell. Published 2011 by John Wiley & Sons Ltd.
© 2011 John Wiley & Sons Ltd.

Clonorchis and *Opisthorchis* liver flukes are parasitic flatworms; as their name implies they are flat and are lancet shaped. The adults live in the bile duct or, less commonly, the pancreatic duct or gall bladder of humans and other mammals[5]. *O. viverrini* is about 7 mm long and 1.5 mm wide, while *C. sinensis* is a little larger[6]. They are hermaphrodites with each worm containing both ovaries and testes (monoecious). The worms are capable of self-fertilization, allowing propagation when worm numbers are low.

Transmission[7]

The life cycle is similar to that of schistosomes, but is more complex, with two intermediate hosts. Eggs are excreted in the faeces of the host – when these come into contact with fresh water they remain dormant until ingested by a snail, at which time the eggs hatch and undergo an asexual reproductive cycle within the snail. Free-swimming cercariae are released but, unlike schistosomes, these do not penetrate the skin of the definitive host; they enter and encyst in the flesh of freshwater fish. The definitive mammalian host is infected by ingesting raw (or inadequately cooked) infected fish. Unfortunately, in many areas where they are endemic there is a deeply culturally entrenched practice of eating raw fish dishes[7]. In the mammalian host they excyst in the duodenum and then pass through the ampulla of Vater into the biliary tree, where they lodge and complete their maturation[6]. Mature worms can survive for at least 25 years; worms were found at autopsy in the biliary tree of a Chinese man who had not visited an endemic area for 26 years[8].

In almost all cases there is local inflammation, while around 10% of patients will develop acute illness; acute symptomatic disease is least commonly seen in those infected with *O. viverrini*, which is the species most often associated with malignant progression.

Both flukes are found mainly in South-East Asia, although their geographical distribution is not identical. *Opisthorchis felineus*, a related species, is found in the Russian Federation and Eastern Europe; it is currently deemed unclassifiable as to carcinogenicity in humans[5]. It is possible that *O. felineus* is not a significant carcinogen because the infected population lack high levels of exposures to dietary cofactors seen in the South-East Asian populations. Diagnosis of fluke infestation is made by detection of parasite eggs in stool samples; even experts may have difficulty in distinguishing *O. viverrini* and *O. felineus* ova, which may complicate differential diagnosis. Fortunately, a good history of potential routes of infection will usually make the distinction, and in any case the treatment is identical; the parasites can usually be eradicated by a short (1-day) course of praziquantel[9].

Transmission of infection is not a risk outwith the endemic areas; this can only occur where this is a confluence of the presence of intermediate host species and the practice of eating raw or poorly cooked fish.

Associated malignancies

Cholangiocarcinoma

The IARC classifies liver flukes as:

■ Group 1 – definitely carcinogenic to humans
  o *O. viverrini*
  o *C. sinensis*
■ Group 3 – not classifiable as to its carcinogenicity to humans
  o *O. felineus*

Cholangiocarcinoma is the only cancer unequivocally linked to liver fluke infection[5]. It is the second commonest primary liver cancer; there are two forms – intrahepatic and extrahepatic[10]. Incidence and mortality for intrahepatic cholangiocarcinoma (ICC) are reported to be rising globally, while those for extrahepatic cholangiocarcinoma (ECC) are falling[11]. The reasons for this are unknown, but the biology of liver fluke infestation precludes this playing any significant role.

The mechanism of fluke-induced cholangiocarcinoma is complex, but it is clear that inflammation plays a major role[9,12,13]. The diet of raw fish which is common in areas of endemicity for fluke infection are also thought to lead to high levels of nitrosamines which are known carcinogens[7]. There is also evidence that liver fluke infection increases levels of production of endogenous nitrosamines[14,15]. The liver fluke may also produce metabolic products which directly stimulate malignant transformation[16-18].

Prevention

Various schemes have been implemented to address the high endemicity of cholangiocarcinoma in areas where liver fluke infection is endemic, These have had limited success to date; it is difficult to introduce hygienic waste disposal where local populations see no alternatives, attempts to change dietary practices have run up against entrenched cultural norms[7]. Localized schemes using prophylactic treatment with praziquantel have had some limited success[19,20] but this carries the risk of inducing chemotherapy resistance[21].

Cholangiocarcinoma is the only cancer unequivocally linked to liver fluke infection[5]. It is the second commonest primary liver cancer; there are two forms – intrahepatic and extrahepatic[10]. Intrahepatic cholangiocarcinoma (ICC) mortality is rising globally, while that for extrahepatic cholangiocarcinoma (ECC) is stable, or possibly decreasing[22,23]. The increasing incidence of ICC cannot be linked to liver fluke infestation, as the parasites cannot be transmitted outwith the known endemic areas areas due to the absence of their obligate intermediate host.

Fluke-related cholangiocarcinoma is exclusively present in those areas in which there is both fluke endemicity and presence of the intermediate host species.

Summary

- Liver flukes are members of the trematode family
- Two species of liver flukes are classed as carcinogens by IARC and for one species the evidence is equivocal
  - O. viverrini   Group 1 (definite carcinogen)
  - C. sinensis   Group 1 (definite carcinogen)
  - O. viverrini   Group 3 (not classifiable)
- Liver fluke infection is associated with cholangiocarcinoma
- Liver flukes do not occur naturally and cannot be transmitted in Europe
  - Intermediate hosts are absent
  - Animal species are found throughout the world, but are not transmissible to humans
- Common throughout South-East Asia and cause serious disease burden

Liver fluke intermediate hosts are absent from Britain (and Western Europe) so all infestations are acquired during travel in endemic regions. The flukes cannot pass directly from mammalian host to mammalian host. Liver fluke infestations, and associated cancers, are rare in the UK; the principal knowledge requirement is for healthcare professionals advising travellers on the precautions needed in endemic areas. The flukes can persist for decades in infected individuals, so a detailed travel history should be taken in any case where there is even a possibility of exposure. There have been isolated incidences of infection acquired from imported contaminated foodstuffs; this means that an absence of travel in endemic areas cannot totally exclude the diagnosis.

References

1. Sripa, B. (2008) Concerted action is needed to tackle liver fluke infections in Asia. *PLoS Neglected Tropical Diseases*, **2**, e232.

2. Lerman, D., Barrett-Connor, E. & Norcross, W. (1982) Intestinal parasites in asymptomatic adult Southeast Asian immigrants. *Journal of Family Practice*, **15**, 443–446.

3. Yossepowitch, O., Gotesman, T., Assous, M., Marva, E., Zimlichman, R. & Dan, M. (2004) Opisthorchiasis from imported raw fish. *Emerging Infectious Diseases*, **10**, 2122–2126.

4. Kaewkes, S. (2003) Taxonomy and biology of liver flukes. *Acta Tropica*, **88**, 177–186.

5. IARC (1994) Schistosomes, liver flukes and *Helicobacter pylori*. IARC Working Group on the evaluation of carcinogenic risks to humans. Lyon, 7–14 June 1994. *IARC Monographs on the Evaluation of Carcinogenic Risks to Humans*, 61, 1–241.

6. Thamavit, W., Shirai, T. & Ito, N. (1999) Liver flukes and biliary cancer. In: *Microbes and Malignancy: Infection as a Cause of Human Cancers* (ed. J. Parsonnet), pp. 346–371. Oxford University Press, Oxford.

7. Sripa, B., Kaewkes, S., Sithithaworn, P., *et al.* (2007) Liver fluke induces cholangiocarcinoma. *PLoS Medicine*, **4**, e201.

8. Attwood, H.D. & Chou, S.T. (1978) The longevity of *Clonorchis sinensis*. *Pathology*, **10**, 153–156.

9. Parkin, D.M., Ohshima, H., Srivatanakul, P. & Vatanasapt, V. (1993) Cholangiocarcinoma: Epidemiology, mechanisms of carcinogenesis and prevention. *Cancer Epidemiology Biomarkers & Prevention*, **2**, 537–544.

10. Khan, S.A., Thomas, H.C., Davidson, B.R. & Taylor-Robinson, S.D. (2005) Cholangiocarcinoma. *Lancet*, **366**, 1303–1314.

11. Khan, S.A., Toledano, M.B. & Taylor-Robinson, S.D. (2008) Epidemiology, risk factors, and pathogenesis of cholangiocarcinoma. *HPB (Oxford)*, **10**, 77–82.

12. Berthiaume, E.P. & Wands, J. (2004) The molecular pathogenesis of cholangiocarcinoma. *Seminars in Liver Diseases*, **24**, 127–137.

13. Blechacz, B. & Gores, G.J. (2008) Cholangiocarcinoma: Advances in pathogenesis, diagnosis, and treatment. *Hepatology*, **48**, 308–321.

14. Srianujata, S., Tonbuth, S., Bunyaratvej, S., Valyasevi, A., Promvanit, N. & Chaivatsagul, W. (1987) High urinary excretion of nitrate and N-nitrosoproline in opisthorchiasis subjects. *IARC Scientific Publications*, **84**, 544–546.

15. Srivatanakul, P., Ohshima, H., Khlat, M., *et al.* (1991) *Opisthorchis viverrini* infestation and endogenous nitrosamines as risk factors for cholangiocarcinoma in Thailand. *International Journal of Cancer*, **48**, 821–825.

16. Thuwajit, C., Thuwajit, P., Kaewkes, S., *et al.* (2004) Increased cell proliferation of mouse fibroblast NIH-3T3 in vitro induced by excretory/secretory product(s) from *Opisthorchis viverrini*. *Parasitology*, **129**, 455–464.

17. Thuwajit, C., Thuwajit, P., Uchida, K., *et al.* (2006) Gene expression profiling defined pathways correlated with fibroblast cell proliferation induced by *Opisthorchis viverrini* excretory/secretory product. *World Journal of Gastroenterology*, **12**, 3585–3592.

18. Harinasuta, T., Riganti, M. & Bunnag, D. (1984) *Opisthorchis viverrini* infection: Pathogenesis and clinical features. *Arzneimittelforschung*, **34**, 1167–1169.

19. Jongsuksuntigul, P. & Imsomboon, T. (1998) Epidemiology of opisthorchiasis and national control program in Thailand. *Southeast Asian Journal of Tropical Medicine and Public Health*, **29**, 327–332.

20. Sithithaworn, P., Haswell-Elkins, M.R., Mairiang, P., *et al.* (1994) Parasite-associated morbidity: Liver fluke infection and bile duct cancer in northeast Thailand. *International Journal of Parasitology*, **24**, 833–843.

21. World Health Organization Regional Office for the Western Pacific. (2002) *Report on the Joint WHO/FAO Workshop on Food-borne Trematode Infections in Asia*, Ha Noi, Vietnam, 26–28 November 2002. World Health Organization Regional Office for the Western Pacific, Manila, Philippines.

22. Taylor-Robinson, S.D., Toledano, M.B., Arora, S., *et al.* (2001) Increase in mortality rates from intrahepatic cholangiocarcinoma in England and Wales 1968–1998. *Gut*, **48**, 816–820.

23. Patel, T. (2001) Increasing incidence and mortality of primary intrahepatic cholangiocarcinoma in the United States. *Hepatology*, **33**, 1353–1357.

14 Unconfirmed associations

There are a number of cancers for which an infectious cause has been suggested but where this is not widely accepted. Some of these have already been alluded to in earlier chapters. This chapter briefly mentions some of those not already discussed and offers references for further reading. They will not be discussed in detail.

Breast cancer

For over 70 years, it has been known that a non-chromosomal factor is involved in the familial patterns observed for murine mammary tumours, and that this could be transmitted in milk[1,2]. The agent responsible in mice has been identified and characterized, and is called the murine mammary tumour virus (MMTV)[3,4].

There has been speculation that human breast cancer may, at least in some cases, be virally induced[5-13]. Both EBV and a human homologue of MMTV have been proposed as causal factors. The evidence is contradictory; at present there is no infectious agent which has been classified by International Agency for Research on Cancer (IARC) as a cause of breast cancer.

Colon cancer

It has been suggested that gut flora may produce carcinogenic metabolites which may in turn be a causal factor of colon cancer[14]; on the basis of studies in experimentally immunosuppressed mice, it has been proposed that the parasitic protozoa ctyptosporidium may induce colon cancer in immunosuppressed humans[15]. There is currently no IARC recognized infectious cause of colon cancer.

Prostate cancer

There is controversy about what, if any, causal contribution infections make to prostate cancer risk. A recent US study concluded, '*This large prospective study of prostate cancer shows no consistent association with specific STIs and a borderline association*

Infectious Causes of Cancer, first edition. By Ken Campbell. Published 2011 by John Wiley & Sons Ltd.
© 2011 John Wiley & Sons Ltd.

with any versus none'[16]; a 2010 US study[17] found an association between sexually transmitted infection (STI), prostatitis and prostate cancer, leaving this an open question. A 2007 study[18] which included the STI *Chlamydia trachomatis*, high-risk HPV strains and HHV-8 found no increased risk for any of these and a previously unreported inverse association between HHV-8 seropositivity and prostate cancer. A persuasive argument against a significant viral contribution is the absence of any HIV-associated increase in prostate cancer incidence[19], although one US study[20] reported duration of HIV-positive status to be associated with increased prostate cancer and proposed that with extended survival an excess of prostate cancer may emerge within the HIV-positive population.

The most plausible mechanism by which infection might increase prostate cancer risk would be the well-recognized sequence of chronic inflammation (prostatitis) leading to increased cell turnover and thus raising the cancer risk. Both prostatitis and prostate cancer are very common in the older male population, which is likely to make it difficult to elucidate causal factors.

Currently, there are no infectious agents recognized by IARC as causes of prostate cancer.

Extra-nodal NHL

Certain viral infections are well established as causing lymphoma, both Hodgkin's and non-Hodgkin's[21-29]. Infection with the bacterium *Helicobacter pylori* is well established as a causal agent for gastric mucosa-associated lymphoid tissue (MALT) lymphoma. A common pathway in MALT NHL appears to be chronic inflammation inducing lymphocyte aggregation[30].

There are other proposed causal links that are not well established, although there is suggestive evidence. One of these is between infection with certain Chlamydiae species, and specific forms of extra-nodal NHL Chlamydiae are obligate intracellular bacteria which are found in eukaryotic cells[31]. *Chlamydia psittaci* is a species which normally infects birds; it is the causal agent in humans of psittacosis (bird-fancier's lung). Infection with *C. psittaci* has been associated with MALT NHL of the ocular adnexa (the structures adjacent to the eye, including eyelids, ocular muscles, etc.), the evidence has recently been reviewed[32]. Other reported associations are between *Campylobacter jejuni* and small intestine MALT NHL and between *Borrelia afzelii* and cutaneous MALT NHL[30].

Lung cancer

Both viral (HPV) and bacterial (*Chlamydophilia pneumoniae*) infections have been proposed as risk factors for lung adenocarcinoma[33-36]. Neither of these is currently recognized by IARC as a causal agent for lung cancer. It is beyond doubt that the primary causal factor for lung cancer is exposure to tobacco smoke, and that this is, and will continue to be, the most important target for reduction in incidence[37].

Summary

Various associations have been reported between infectious agents and specific malignancy for which the evidence falls short of demonstrating causality. In some cases, such as breast cancer, a strong argument for an infectious link is analogy from murine mammary tumours which are known to be caused by a specific virus. In others, such as extra-nodal NHL, the biology of the malignancy is highly consistent with an infectious aetiology and there are multiple candidates; of these, only *H. pylori* is a proven carcinogen, being associated with certain forms of stomach cancer. It is highly plausible that further infectious causes of cancer will be identified.

References

1. Roscoe B. Jackson Memorial Laboratory Staff (1933) The existence of non-chromosomal influence in the incidence of mammary tumors in mice. *Science*, **78**, 465–466.
2. Bittner, J.J. (1936) Some possible effects of nursing on the mammary gland tumor incidence in mice. *Science*, **84**, 162.
3. Bryan, W.R., Kahler, H., Shimkin, M.B. & Andervont, H.B. (1942) Extraction and ultracentrifugation of mammary tumor inciter of mice. *Journal of the National Cancer Institute*, **2**, 451.
4. Visscher, M.B., Green, R.G. & Bittner, J. (1942) Characterization of milk influence in spontaneous mammary carcinoma. *Proceedings of the Society for Experimental Biology and Medicine*, **49**, 94–96.
5. Herrmann, K. & Niedobitek, G. (2003) Lack of evidence for an association of Epstein-Barr virus infection with breast carcinoma. *Breast Cancer Research*, **5**, R13–R17.
6. Indik, S., Gunzburg, W.H., Kulich, P., Salmons, B. & Rouault, F. (2007) Rapid spread of mouse mammary tumor virus in cultured human breast cells. *Retrovirology*, **4**, 73.
7. Kleer, C.G., Tseng, M.D., Gutsch, D.E., *et al.* (2002) Detection of Epstein-Barr virus in rapidly growing fibroadenomas of the breast in immunosuppressed hosts. *Modern Pathology*, **15**, 759–764.
8. Lau, S.K., Chen, Y.Y., Berry, G.J., Yousem, S.A. & Weiss, L.M. (2003) Epstein-Barr virus infection is not associated with fibroadenomas of the breast in immunosuppressed patients after organ transplantation. *Modern Pathology*, **16**, 1242–1247.
9. Lawson, J.S., Tran, D. & Rawlinson, W.D. (2001) From Bittner to Barr: A viral, diet and hormone breast cancer aetiology hypothesis. *Breast Cancer Research*, **3**, 81–85.
10. Lawson, J.S., Tran, D.D., Carpenter, E., *et al.* (2006) Presence of mouse mammary tumour-like virus gene sequences may be associated with morphology of specific human breast cancer. *Journal of Clinical Pathology*, **59**, 1287–1292.
11. Thompson, M.P. & Kurzrock, R. (2004) Epstein-Barr virus and cancer. *Clinical Cancer Research*, **10**, 803–821.
12. Yasui, Y., Potter, J.D., Stanford, J.L., *et al.* (2001) Breast cancer risk and "delayed" primary Epstein-Barr virus infection. *Cancer Epidemiology, Biomarkers & Prevention*, **10**, 9–16.
13. Melana, S.M., Nepomnaschy, I., Hasa, J., *et al.* (2010) Detection of human mammary tumor virus proteins in human breast cancer cells. *Journal of Virological Methods*, **163**, 157–161.
14. Parsonnet, J. (1995) Bacterial infection as a cause of cancer. *Environmental Health Perspectives*, **103** (Suppl. 8), 263–268.

15. Certad, G., Ngouanesavanh, T., Guyot, K., *et al.* (2007) *Cryptosporidium parvum*, a potential cause of colic adenocarcinoma. *Infectious Agents and Cancer*, **2**, 22.

16. Huang, W.Y., Hayes, R., Pfeiffer, R., *et al.* (2008) Sexually transmissible infections and prostate cancer risk. *Cancer Epidemiology, Biomarkers & Prevention*, **17**, 2374–2381.

17. Cheng, I., Witte, J.S., Jacobson, S.J., *et al.* (2010) Prostatitis, sexually transmitted diseases, and prostate cancer: The California Men's Health Study. *PLoS One*, **5**, e8736.

18. Sutcliffe, S., Giovannucci, E., Gaydos, C.A., *et al.* (2007) Plasma antibodies against *Chlamydia trachomatis*, human papillomavirus, and human herpesvirus type 8 in relation to prostate cancer: A prospective study. *Cancer Epidemiology, Biomarkers & Prevention*, **16**, 1573–1580.

19. Boshoff, C. & Weiss, R. (2002) AIDS-related malignancies. *Nature Reviews Cancer*, **2**, 373–382.

20. Crum, N.F., Spencer, C.R. & Amling, C.L. (2004) Prostate carcinoma among men with human immunodeficiency virus infection. *Cancer*, **101**, 294–299.

21. Kuppers, R. (2009) The biology of Hodgkin's lymphoma. *Nature Reviews Cancer*, **9**, 15–27.

22. Diehl, V., Thomas, R.K. & Re, D. (2004) Part II: Hodgkin's lymphoma – Diagnosis and treatment. *Lancet Oncology*, **5**, 19–26.

23. Hennessy, B.T., Hanrahan, E.O. & Daly, P.A. (2004) Non-Hodgkin lymphoma: An update. *Lancet Oncology*, **5**, 341–353.

24. Isaacson, P.G. & Du, M.Q. (2004) MALT lymphoma: From morphology to molecules. *Nature Reviews Cancer*, **4**, 644–653.

25. Thomas, R.K., Re, D., Wolf, J. & Diehl, V. (2004) Part I: Hodgkin's lymphoma – Molecular biology of Hodgkin and Reed-Sternberg cells. *Lancet Oncology*, **5**, 11–18.

26. van den Bosch, C.A. (2004) Is endemic Burkitt's lymphoma an alliance between three infections and a tumour promoter? *Lancet Oncology*, **5**, 738–746.

27. Young, L.S. & Rickinson, A.B. (2004) Epstein-Barr virus: 40 years on. *Nature Reviews Cancer*, **4**, 757–768.

28. Carbone, A. (2003) Emerging pathways in the development of AIDS-related lymphomas. *Lancet Oncology*, **4**, 22–29.

29. Yeo, W., Hui, P., Chow, J.H. & Mok, T.S. (2001) Hepatocellular carcinoma and lymphoma – two hepatitis B virus-related malignant diseases. *Lancet Oncology*, **2**, 543.

30. Engels, E.A. (2007) Infectious agents as causes of non-Hodgkin lymphoma. *Cancer Epidemiology, Biomarkers & Prevention*, **16**, 401–404.

31. Peeling, R.W. & Brunham, R.C. (1996) Chlamydiae as pathogens: New species and new issues. *Emerging Infectious Diseases*, **2**, 307–319.

32. Decaudin, D., de Cremoux, P., Vincent-Salomon, A., Dendale, R. & Rouic, L.L. (2006) Ocular adnexal lymphoma: A review of clinicopathologic features and treatment options. *Blood*, **108**, 1451–1460.

33. Chen, Y.C., Chen, J.H., Richard, K., Chen, P.Y. & Christiani, D.C. (2004) Lung adenocarcinoma and human papillomavirus infection. *Cancer*, **101**, 1428–1436.

34. Chiou, H.L., Wu, M.F., Liaw, Y.C., *et al.* (2003) The presence of human papillomavirus type 16/18 DNA in blood circulation may act as a risk marker of lung cancer in Taiwan. *Cancer*, **97**, 1558–1563.

35. Kocazeybek, B. (2003) Chronic *Chlamydophila pneumoniae* infection in lung cancer, a risk factor: A case-control study. *Journal of Medical Microbiology*, **52**, 721–726.

36. Littman, A.J., White, E., Jackson, L.A., *et al.* (2004) *Chlamydia pneumoniae* infection and risk of lung cancer. *Cancer Epidemiology, Biomarkers & Prevention*, **13**, 1624–1630.

37. Boyle, P & Levin, B. (eds) (2008) Lung cancer. In: *World Cancer Report 2008*, pp. 390–395. International Agency for Research on Cancer, Lyon.

Summary Tables

Herpesviruses

Organism	**Epstein–Barr virus**
Synonyms	EBV, HHV-4
Natural host(s)	Human
Description	Gamma-1 herpesvirus
Special features	Establishes life-long latency
Epidemiology of infection	Global population ~ ubiquitous
Mode(s) of transmission	Intimate non-sexual contact, especially kissing.
Cancer(s) associated (International Agency for Research on Cancer [IARC] carcinogen category)	IARC Group 1 (definitely carcinogenic in humans); • Burkitt's lymphoma • Sinonasal angiocentric T-cell lymphoma • Immunosuppression-related lymphoma • Hodgkin's disease • Nasopharyngeal carcinoma. Not listed by IARC but some cases reported as EBV-positive; • Breast cancer • Gastric cancer • Leiomyosarcoma in immunosuppressed patients
Cofactors	Any form of immunosuppression Burkitt's – malaria, HIV Other NHL – HIV, iatrogenic

Other associated diseases	NPC – genetic susceptibility, dietary carcinogens
	 • Infectious mononucleosis (glandular fever),
	 • Diseases associated with X-linked lymphoproliferation and other congenital immunodeficiencies
	     o Overwhelming lymphoproliferative syndrome (fatal infectious mononucleosis)
	     o Hypogammaglobulinaemia
	 • Diseases in acquired immunodeficiency and after transplantation
	     o Polyclonal lymphoproliferation
	     o Chronic Epstein-Barr virus infection

Potential prevention strategies	EBV vaccination Elimination of co-factors

Organism	**Human herpes virus 8**
Synonyms	Kaposi Sarcoma-associated herpes virus, HHV8, KSHV
Natural host(s)	Humans
Description	Gamma-2 herpesvirus
Special features	The only human herpesvirus with a geographically restricted distribution
Epidemiology of infection	Global population – geographically restricted distribution – 'the vious is prevalent in Africa in Mediterranean countries, among Jews and Arabs and certain Amerindians'
Mode(s) of transmission	Uncertain sexual transmission? saliva (mother to child, sib to sib)?
Cancer(s) associated (IARC carcinogen category)	Kaposi's sarcoma (Gp 2a, probably carcinogenic) '*There is compelling but as yet limited evidence for a role of KSHV/HHV8 in the causation of Kaposi's sarcoma*'
Cofactors	Immunosuppression (incl. HIV infection), podoconiosis
Other associated diseases	Primary effusion lymphoma, multi-centric Castleman's disease
Potential prevention strategies	No vaccine available. Route of transmission unclear therefore no obvious scope for health education

Hepatitis Viruses

Organism	**Hepatitis B virus**
Synonyms	HBV, Hep B
Natural host(s)	Humans – closely related species found in many mammals
Description	DNA virus – partially double-stranded circular genome. Eight known genotypes – vary in geographical distribution and in risk of chronic disease and of cancer
Special features	Minimally cytopathic; outcome of acute infection depends on age at time of infection and on intensity of immune response
Epidemiology of infection	Global population ~ one-third Perinatal infection common in developing world; later (adult) infection common in developed world
Mode(s) of transmission	Infants – perinatal, exposure to infectious maternal body-fluids Childhood – intimate non-sexual contact Adult – IV drug abuse, sexually transmitted, iatrogenic (rare in West)
Cancer(s) associated (IARC carcinogen category)	Group 1 (definitely carcinogenic in humans). • Hepatocellular carcinoma
Cofactors	High alcohol intake, HBC co-infection, aflatoxin
Other associated diseases	Hepatitis (acute or chronic), cirrhosis
Potential prevention strategies	Vaccination, health education, risk reduction strategies for drug users

Organism	**Hepatitis C virus**
Synonyms	Hepacvirus, Hep C
Natural host(s)	Humans – closely related species found in many mammals
Description	RNA virus
Special features	Minimally cytopathic, family Flaviridae. Excites strong immune response but can evade both innate and adaptive immune systems
Epidemiology of infection	Global population ~ 2% ~ 123 million people Infection is more common in developed world
Mode(s) of transmission	Infants – perinatal, exposure to infectious maternal body-fluids Childhood – intimate non-sexual contact Adult – IV drug abuse, iatrogenic (rare in West)
Cancer(s) associated (IARC carcinogen category)	*Group* – 1 (definitely carcinogenic in humans). • Hepatocellular carcinoma • Non-Hodgkin lymphoma*
Cofactors	Alcohol, HBV and/or HIV co-infection, betel nut chewing
Other associated diseases	Hepatitis, cirrhosis
Potential prevention strategies	Vaccination – no vaccine yet available Public health education Risk reduction programs in prisons and among drug users

* In a review published in 2009 of carcinogenicity of biological agents, IARC declared that infection with HCV can cause NHL. This will be formally included in part B of volume 100 of the IARC monographs.

Papillomaviruses

Organism	**Human papillomavirus**
Synonyms	HPV
Natural host(s)	Humans
Description	DNA virus of papovavirus family
Special features	Overwhelming majority of infections rapidly resolve without treatment
Epidemiology of infection	Global population ~ Ubiquitous; estimated that over 80% of sexually active individuals will be infected at some time
Mode(s) of transmission	Sexual Intimate non-sexual contact
Cancer(s) associated (IARC carcinogen category)	IARC Group 1 (definitely carcinogenic in humans); • Cervical cancer (HPV 16, 18, 31, 33, 35, 39, 45, 51, 52, 56, 58, 59, 66) • Vulva, vagina, penis, anus, oral cavity, oropharynx (HPV 16) • Skin (squamous-cell carcinoma) in patients with epidermodysplasia verruciformis (HPV genus-beta types 5 & 8) IARC Group 2B (possibly carcinogenic in humans) • Larynx and periungual skin (squamous-cell carcinoma) (HPV 16) • Vulva, vagina, penis, anus, oral cavity and larynx (HPV 18) • Larynx (squamous-cell carcinoma), vulva, penis, anus (HPV 6, 11) • Skin (squamous-cell carcinoma), (HPV genus-beta types) Conjunctiva (squamous-cell carcinoma)
Cofactors	Smoking High parity Co-infection (including HSV and HIV)
Other associated diseases	Low oncogenicity strains cause warts (genital and cutaneous)
Potential prevention strategies	HPV vaccination – limited number of strains Secondary prevention of cervical cancer by screening for pre-malignant lesions

Retroviruses

Organism	**Human T-lymphotropic virus**
Synonyms	Human T-cell Leukaemia Virus, HTLV
Natural host(s)	Humans
Description	Two strains, HTLV-I and HTLV-II
Special features	Only known human oncornaviridae Extreme latency – up to 4 decades from infection to cancer
Epidemiology of infection	Global population ~ HTLV-I 15–20 million HTLV-II unknown
Mode(s) of transmission	Mother to child – especially breast-feeding beyond 6/12 Sexual transmission Blood-borne – transfusion/i.v. drug use
Cancer(s) associated (IARC carcinogen category)	IARC Group 1 (definitely carcinogenic in humans) • Adult T-cell leukaemia/lymphoma (HTLV-I) HTLV-II is Group 3 (not classifiable as to carcinogenicity in humans)
Cofactors	Stronglyoides infection – shortens lag from infection to malignancy by up to 30 years
Other associated diseases	HTLV-1-associated myelopathy/ Tropical spastic paresis (HAM/TSP) Uveitis (in endemic areas) Arthropathy?
Potential prevention strategies	Block transmission – modification of breast-feeding practices in high-risk areas, risk reduction strategies for drug users Screening of blood for transfusion

Organism	**Human immunodeficiency virus**
Synonyms	*HIV-1, HIV-2*
Natural host(s)	Man
Description	Highly variable retrovirus
Special features	Suppresses immune system Anatomical reservoir unknown
Epidemiology of infection	Global population ~ almost 60 million
Mode(s) of transmission	Sexual transmission, blood-borne, vertical transmission during pregnancy and childbirth
Cancer(s) associated (IARC carcinogen category)	HIV01 – Group 1 (definitely carcinogenic in humans) HIV-2 – Group 2B (possibly carcinogenic in humans)
Cofactors	Other STDs, malnutrition
Other associated diseases	See CDC classification of AIDS-defining and non AIDS-defining associated conditions[1]
Potential prevention strategies	Vaccination – on effective vaccine currently available Health education Interventions to block vertical transmission

Polyomaviruses

Organism	**Simian Virus 40**
Synonyms	*SV40*
Natural host(s)	Monkeys
Description	Small DNA virus
Special features	Believed to have entered human population as contaminant of polio vaccine Status as human carcinogen highly controversial Evidence for onward transmission in humans equivocal
Epidemiology of infection	Global population ~ Unknown, hundreds of millions believed exposed to infected vaccine
Mode(s) of transmission	May be sporadic cross-species infection from wild monkeys Major route of entry to human population – contaminated polio vaccine No definite evidence of horizontal or vertical spread in human population
Cancer(s) associated (IARC carcinogen category)	Not reviewed by IARC
Cofactors	None known
Other associated diseases	None in humans
Potential prevention strategies	N/A

Organism	**Merkel cell polyomavirus**
Synonyms	*MCV, MCPV*
Natural host(s)	?
Description	A newly discovered polyomavirus
Special features	Discovered in 2008 Associated with Merkel cell carcinoma, a rare highly-lethal skin cancer
Epidemiology of infection	Global population ~ highly speculative reports suggest up to 1 billion people infected
Mode(s) of transmission	Unknown
Cancer(s) associated (IARC carcinogen category)	No IARC assessment
Cofactors	Not known
Other associated diseases	None confirmed May be associated with polyomavirus nephropathy and/or progressive multi-focal leukoencephalopathy
Potential prevention strategies	Possibly vaccination – no polyomavirus vaccines are currently available

Helicobacter pylori

Organism	***Helicobacter pylori***
Synonyms	*Campylobacter pylorus, Campylobacter pylori*
Natural host(s)	Humans – closely related species found in many mammals
Description	Gram-negative, flagellated, spiral bacterium about 0.5 µm × 3.0 µm
Special features	Only micro-organism which can colonize stomach; survives acidic gastric environment by urease catalysis of urea to release ammonia and carbon dioxide and by tunnelling into the protective mucous layer covering gastric epithelium
Epidemiology of infection	Global population ~ 50% Varies from 30% (Western Europe) to 90% (Asia) Falling rates over time in developed world
Mode(s) of transmission	Oral-oral or faecal-oral with parents or siblings being principle sources of exposure Possibly contaminated water supplies
Cancer(s) associated (IARC carcinogen category)	IARC Group 1 (definitely carcinogenic in humans); Gastric adenocarcinoma (non-cardia) Gastric mucosal-associated tissue lymphoma (MALToma) No IARC classification but reported causal link Pancreatic cancer The following tumours are reported as being less common in the presence of *H. pylori* infection Gastric adenocarcinoma (cardia) Oesophageal cancer
Cofactors	Diet – high in salt, smoked meat and fish, low in fresh fruit and vegetables; bile reflux syndromes; smoking; high alcohol
Other associated diseases	Chronic gastritis Peptic ulcer
Potential prevention strategies	Eradication of *H. pylori* by improved sanitation Eradication of *H. pylori* by vaccination Elimination of *H. pylori* by antibiotic therapy Screening at-risk populations for *H. pylori* infection

Schistosomes

Organism	***Schistosoma haematobium***
Synonyms	Bilharzia
Natural host(s)	Definitive – human Intermediate – freshwater snails
Description	Trematode flatworms
Special features	Most prevalent form globally, about 85% of cases in sub-Saharan Africa
Epidemiology of infection	Global population ~ over 100 million
Mode(s) of transmission	Intermediate hosts are infected following contamination of still or running fresh water by human urine containing eggs; infected snails release intermediate forms (cercariae) into water; cercariae can penetrate human skin, these migrate to veins draining the urinary bladder where they mature into adult forms
Cancer(s) associated (IARC carcinogen category)	IARC Group 1 (definitely carcinogenic in humans); • Urinary bladder carcinoma
Cofactors	Exposure to certain chemicals and smoking are independent risk factors for bladder cancer
Other associated diseases	Acute schistosomiasis, anaemia, bladder inflammatory disease, granulomas (from parasite eggs), renal malfunction, genital schistosomiasis, developmental impairment. Illness arising from schistosomal infection is known as bilharzia, which was recognized clinically centuries before the parasite was discovered.
Potential prevention strategies	Primary prevention requires scrupulous avoidance of contact with contaminated water and, at a population level, sanitary disposal of urine and faeces. Secondary prevention involves recognition of infection and treatment (with praziquantel) to eliminate infection before chronic inflammation is induced.

Liver Flukes

Organism	***Clonorchis sinensis***
Synonyms	Liver fluke, trematode
Natural host(s)	Definitive – humans, other mammals Intermediate – (1) freshwater snails (2) freshwater fish
Description	Multicellular parasite with a complex lifecycle involving two intermediate hosts
Special features	More likely than other flukes to cause bile duct and gall bladder stones
Epidemiology of infection	Global population ~ 600 million at risk Infected population ~ estimated 7 million
Mode(s) of transmission	Intermediate hosts are infected following contamination of still or running fresh water by human waste and infection of humans occurs by eating raw or inadequately cooked fish.
Cancer(s) associated (IARC carcinogen category)	Group 1 (definitely carcinogenic in humans) Cholangiocarcinoma
Cofactors	High salt intake Nitrosamines ingested in raw fish dishes
Other associated diseases	Gall bladder inflammation – probably a significant factor in carcinogenesis (by analogy with cirrhosis and HCC)
Potential prevention strategies	Theoretically easy to prevent by thorough cooking of fish before consumption but entrenched cultural norms have frustrated this in practice

Organism	***Opisthorchis viverrini***
Synonyms	Liver fluke, trematode
Natural host(s)	Definitive – humans, other mammals Intermediate – (1) freshwater snails (2) freshwater fish
Description	Multicellular parasite with complex life style involving two intermediate hosts
Special features	Exceptionally high incidence in some areas of north-east Thailand, where at least one-third of the population is infected
Epidemiology of infection	Global population ~ estimated at 9 million
Mode(s) of transmission	Intermediate hosts are infected following contamination of still or running fresh water by human waste and infection of humans occurs by eating raw or inadequately cooked fish.
Cancer(s) associated (IARC carcinogen category)	Group 1 (definitely carcinogenic in humans) Cholangiocarcinoma
Cofactors	High salt intake Nitrosamines ingested in raw fish dishes
Other associated diseases	Gall bladder inflammation – probably a significant factor in carcinogenesis (by analogy with cirrhosis and HCC)
Potential prevention strategies	Theoretically easy to prevent by thorough cooking of fish before consumption but entrenched cultural norms have frustrated this in practice

Reference

1. Centers for Disease Control (1993) 1993 Revised classification system for HIV infection and expanded surveillance case definition for AIDS among adolescents and adults. *Morbidity Mortality Weekly Report (MMWR)*, **42**, RR17.

Index

Infectious Causes of Cancer, first edition. By Ken Campbell. Published 2011 by John Wiley & Sons Ltd.
© 2011 John Wiley & Sons Ltd.